Clinical Audit in Physiotherapy:
From Theory into Practice

Clinical Audit in Physiotherapy: From Theory into Practice

Sue Barnard MSc MCSP

Gayle Hartigan

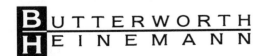

BUTTERWORTH
HEINEMANN

OXFORD BOSTON JOHANNESBURG MELBOURNE NEW DELHI SINGAPORE

Butterworth-Heinemann
Linacre House, Jordan Hill, Oxford OX2 8DP
225 Wildwood Avenue, Woburn, MA 01801-2041
A division of Reed Educational and Professional Publishing Ltd

Ⓡ A member of the Reed Elsevier plc group

First published 1998

© Reed Educational and Professional Publishing Ltd 1998

British Library Cataloguing in Publication Data
A catalogue record for this book is available from the British Library

Library of Congress Cataloguing in Publication Data
A catalogue record for this book is available from the Library of Congress

ISBN 0 7506 3779 X

Printed and bound in Great Britain by Martins the Printers Ltd, Berwick upon Tweed

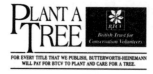

Contents

Preface

This book is designed to complement the many existing books dealing with clinical audit. In this context, it deals specifically with clinical audit and outcome measurement in physiotherapy, and the ways in which physiotherapists participate in clinical audit within the multiprofessional team. Although clinical audit in the National Health Service (NHS) has been around for a decade or so, there remains a paucity of knowledge and experience in some areas and the occasional pocket of distrust. The book places physiotherapy audit into its historical context and converts theory into practice by using real physiotherapy audit examples – warts and all! It is deliberately lightly referenced, preferring to draw from practical (often unpublished) physiotherapy examples and the actual experiences of physiotherapists engaged in clinical audit. Each chapter does, however, conclude with a brief reference section pointing the reader to more academic and specific texts.

Written primarily for physiotherapists embarking upon clinical audit, it is hoped that physiotherapy students will also find this book a useful guide to the principles and practice of physiotherapy audit, and the way in which it fits into the wider clinical audit arena. As the main thrust of clinical audit has been within the NHS, the examples in the book relate, on the whole, to physiotherapy practice within the NHS. The principles, however, are eminently transferable to the private and independent sectors.

The authors would like to thank the following people for their assistance with this book and/or for permission to use the audit examples herein:

Jean Alvis, Physiotherapy Manager, The Royal Bournemouth and Christchurch Hospitals NHS Trust.
Margaret Jater, Physiotherapy Manager, Bassetlaw Hospital and Community Services NHS Trust, Worksop.
John Langridge, Manager, Physiotherapy Services, Southampton University Hospitals NHS Trust.
Bunny le Roux, TELER, Sheffield.
Sue Mawson, Senior Lecturer in Physiotherapy, Sheffield Hallam University.
Judy Mead, Senior Professional Advisor, Chartered Society of Physiotherapy.

Wendy Mills, Physiotherapy Professional Advisor, Portsmouth Healthcare NHS Trust.

Penelope Robinson, Director of Professional Affairs, Chartered Society of Physiotherapy.

Sue Barnard
Gayle Harligan

Introduction

Clinical audit has emerged, over recent years, as a major tool in the development and implementation of strategies to improve the clinical effectiveness of healthcare interventions in the UK. In 1996, published guidance on promoting the improvement of clinical effectiveness, issued to all chief executives of health authorities and NHS trusts by the NHS Executive of the Department of Health (NHSE), stated that clinicians should be able to 'base their routine practice on the best available evidence of effectiveness and . . . systematically to monitor the results of their care, in particular through clinical audit.' (NHSE, 1996).

Clinical audit is a key component in providing evidence of the effectiveness of clinical interventions and is therefore a discrete and important strand of the broader drive towards improving clinical effectiveness in which research and development, evidence-based medicine, outcome measurement and quality assurance also feature. Each strand is inextricably interdependent; for example, published research findings are of little value if there is no mechanism to ensure that they are implemented into routine clinical practice, and a clinical audit project, which sets local standards for an aspect of care, is a pointless exercise if the standards have not been based on accepted evidence of clinical effectiveness.

Although medical audit (which monitored medical practice only) was formally introduced into healthcare in the UK in 1989, followed by nursing and therapies audit in 1990, collectively referred to as 'clinical audit' since 1993, enthusiastic interest in and practical guidance for clinical audit initiatives in physiotherapy have been slow to evolve (for a number of reasons which are explored in detail later in this book), and there exist a number of physiotherapists in the UK who remain personally uninvolved in clinical audit or who participate reluctantly without fully understanding why either their participation or the process itself is required.

The purpose of this book, therefore, is to provide comprehensive and detailed information on all aspects of clinical audit activity in physiotherapy in a straightforward format which is easy to read and digest. It attempts to explain national initiatives in simple language and to interpret some of the more esoteric jargon which has been used to define clinical audit in the past. The major aims are as follows:

1. To set out the rationale behind the introduction of clinical audit as part of the National Health Service reforms and its wider role as a tool to promote improvement of clinical effectiveness.
2. To explore the many uses of clinical audit in physiotherapy and its roles in service evaluation, postgraduate education, continuing professional development, guideline development, clinical benchmarking and accreditation.
3. To give an overview of what the process of clinical audit involves and advice on how physiotherapists can harness the resources and information required to get started.
4. To provide practical guidance on how to introduce clinical audit within a physiotherapy service, including specific examples of previous physiotherapy audits and ideas for future projects.

The book also includes further sources of advice and information on clinical audit issues and a list of useful addresses.

Reference

NHSE (1996). *Promoting Clinical Effectiveness – A Framework for Action In and Through the NHS.* Crown copyright. NHSE, Leeds.

SECTION 1
DEVELOPMENT OF CLINICAL AUDIT IN HEALTHCARE

1
Introduction of clinical audit within the National Health Service

Concept

Clinical audit was introduced in 1989, as part of the National Health Service (NHS) reforms, on the premise that purchasers of healthcare services, within an internal market, would require evidence of the effectiveness of the services purchased and a mechanism to monitor, improve and assure the quality of every aspect of healthcare offered by each provider unit. This premise is considered in greater detail later in this chapter. The concept of audit received its impetus with the publication of the Government's NHS Review Working Paper 6, entitled *Working for Patients*, in which medical (not clinical) audit was described as a systematic method of improving the quality of patient care (Department of Health, 1989).

Official definition

The Department of Health (1993) defined clinical audit as follows:

> Clinical audit involves systematically looking at the procedures used for diagnosis, care and treatment, examining how associated resources are used and investigating the effect care has on the outcome and quality of life for the patient.

The underlying concept is that the end result of the process of clinical audit should be an improvement in the effectiveness and quality of patient care.

The official definition is rather vague in that it sets out the basic principles of audit, i.e. that we should be looking at what we do, keeping an eye on how much it costs and checking whether it does any good, but it offers no guidance on the methods to be adopted and gives no indication whether some areas of clinical practice may be of a higher priority for audit than others. This was not an oversight on the part of the Department of Health; the official definition was left intentionally vague so that the introduction of audit might be regarded as non-prescriptive from the clinical viewpoint (Crombie *et al.*, 1993). It was hoped that clinicians of all professions would feel free to choose audit methods and topics which they deemed most appropriate and to concentrate on areas where they felt specific improvements could be made.

It was agreed at the outset that, if clinical audit was to succeed as more than a paper exercise and to achieve measurable improvements to patient care, the process would have to be professionally led. It was acknowledged that clinical practice could be improved by clinicians only, and that it was the clinicians who were best qualified to identify specific areas of practice which could be improved through audit. Because the success of audit depended not only upon clinical judgement and expertise, but also upon securing the confidence and commitment of the participating clinicians, it was vital that the clinicians should have ownership of the process by which their practice was being audited. It was stipulated that audit results should be anonymous, with active non-identification of both patient and individual clinician, and improvements were to be achieved by 'peer review' which meant the evaluation of a (non-identified) clinician's work by other clinicians in the same profession with comparable training and experience.

These safeguards, which were built into the process of clinical audit to protect and enhance clinical confidence, were often overlooked in the past. For a number of years, suspicion lingered in some quarters that clinical audit was a 'management weapon' used to justify unwelcome cuts, performance review and even the dismantling of some clinical services, rather than a self-regulatory tool to improve the effectiveness of clinical practice, and to enhance clinical education and professional development. The misapprehension was unfortunate and counter-productive, and it remains important to emphasize the value of clinical audit to clinicians.

Rationale

It has been stated that the purpose of clinical audit is to improve the effectiveness of patient care. But, surely, clinicians have always sought ways of improving healthcare, both as part of the commitment to patients and part of individual professional development, so why did this formal process of clinical audit suddenly become necessary? The answer to that question lies within the fundamental changes which have taken place within the NHS since the mid-1980s. Simply, an internal market has been created for healthcare provision, the NHS has become a business, and the patient is now a consumer, on whose behalf local health authorities can 'shop around' for the best services provided, at the best value for the taxpayers' money they are spending.

As in any business which competes for customers in the commercial setting, quality assurance has become all important in the newly reformed

NHS; the new onus is not only to provide quality healthcare services at appropriate cost but to provide evidence to the purchasers of healthcare that the service offered is of high quality and good value for the financial investment. A useful analogy, in commercial terms, would be the 'never knowingly undersold' guarantee of the John Lewis Partnership on the High Street, which assures its customers that they will not find either better quality or lower prices elsewhere.

Quality assurance has become a corporate (central) function of every organization with responsibility for delivering healthcare; it involves setting quality standards for every aspect of service provision and the continuous monitoring of those standards with a view to improving the effectiveness of services wherever possible. Clinical audit is an integral part of the corporate function of quality assurance and is concerned with standard setting, monitoring and making improvements to the effectiveness of the clinical services provided. Therefore, in physiotherapy, clinical audit provides evidence to assure the purchasers of healthcare that physiotherapy is a high quality clinical service which is effective in terms of both the clinical outcome for patients and value for money.

Although its role in the contracting process continues to increase in importance, clinical audit should not be regarded *solely* as a means of marketing quality services to the external purchasers of healthcare. It also has many valuable uses, internally, within a department. For example, the clinical audit process can be used to monitor and improve efficiency in the organization and delivery of local physiotherapy services, which can benefit clinicians as well as patients if it also improves the working environment.

In addition, investigating ways to improve patient care has been a fundamental part of clinical practice, in all professions, since long before the NHS reforms of the 1980s, and the clinical audit process supports such investigation on a systematic basis. Although not a substitute for robust research, clinical audit can provide evidence of the effectiveness of physiotherapy interventions when it is not possible to gather such data in a randomized controlled trial, and review of audit data and results extends and enhances postgraduate physiotherapy education.

Early funding arrangements for audit

It has been stated that medical (not clinical) audit was introduced following publication of the Government's NHS Review Working Paper 6 in 1989 (Department of Health, 1989). Facilitation and development of medical audit were financed using money which had been 'top sliced' from the national budget for healthcare provision, i.e. extracted before the general NHS allocations were made to regional health authorities for healthcare provision, and retained separately in a central fund. Funding for audit was distributed directly to hospitals and trusts on an annual basis and ring-fenced for the first 4 years, which meant, primarily, that it could not be spent on anything other than audit, but also that monies which remained unspent at the end of one financial year could be rolled forward to the next without penalty or reduction of the following year's allocation.

The second stage in the development of clinical audit was the recognition, a year later, that, if the patient was indeed the consumer, then the provision of quality care could not remain the exclusive domain of doctors; audit would have to expand and become applicable to any episode of healthcare provided by any clinical profession. Therefore, in 1990, funding was made available for nursing and therapies audit and this was also ring-fenced for 3 years.

Different funding, different approaches

It has been acknowledged by the Department of Health that, initially, different approaches to clinical audit were adopted by different professions and that these were largely influenced by the funding mechanism, with medical audit funding being allocated directly to hospitals and NHS trusts on the basis of the number of consultants employed, and nursing/therapy audit monies distributed to regional health authorities and allocated to individual departments on a project bidding system (Department of Health, 1994).

As a result, doctors found themselves with the immediate financial resources to pay for computer and administrative support for audit which, in turn, allowed them to develop medical audit programmes which addressed specific areas of clinical practice and effectiveness from the earliest stages, and to develop the educational and professional development aspects of audit. A natural progression was the early incorporation of the requirement to perform medical audit into the employment contracts of doctors, and medical audit is now officially one of the strands upon which accreditation in medicine is dependent.

It is generally recognized that the nursing and therapy professions found it more difficult to obtain funding for clinical audit development and, because of having to bid in open competition against limited funds, early audit activity in the non-medical clinical professions, including physiotherapy, tended to concentrate on organizational issues, non-clinical quality and patient's charter standards.

Changes in funding arrangements for audit

Ring-fenced central funding for medical, nursing and therapies audit ceased in April 1994 and, following devolution of the regional health authorities in 1995/96, funding for audit has been included in the general healthcare allocations to unitary health authorities, of which there were 100 in England, as at 1 April 1996, each covering an average (mean) population of just below 500 000. If we consider that there are approximately 400 provider units offering healthcare services to purchasers, this perhaps illustrates the freedom of choice available to health authorities and the perceived benefits of 'shopping around' for both clinical and cost effectiveness of care.

Specific funding for audit is now written into the service contract between the purchasers (local health authorities and GP fundholders) and providers (NHS hospitals, acute and community trusts) of healthcare. This has resulted in a switch of emphasis and it is the purchasers who now have responsibility, through the contracting process, for the future development and evolution of clinical audit.

A letter from the NHS Executive of the Department of Health in October 1995 set out the new responsibilities of the health authorities with regard to clinical audit and required them both to promote participation in audit by all healthcare professionals and to monitor progress of the continuing development of clinical audit in all professions (NHSE, 1995).

Health authorities have been urged to promote and monitor changes in healthcare delivery through the use of guidelines, clinical audit, postgraduate education, etc. and are charged with the integration of clinical audit across primary and other healthcare sectors (NHSE, 1996).

Informed professional advice and increasingly sophisticated measures of clinical performance and outcome will be required by health authorities in their monitoring and further development of clinical audit, and it is important for physiotherapists to develop their own knowledge base in clinical audit to inform future dialogue with the purchasers of their services.

References

Crombie I.K., Davies H.T.O., Abraham S.C.S., Florey C. du V. (1993). *The Audit Handbook: Improving Health Care Through Clinical Audit*. John Wiley and Sons, Chichester.

Department of Health (1989). *Medical Audit: Working Paper 6 – Working for Patients*. HMSO, London.

Department of Health (1993). *Clinical Audit: Meeting and Improving Standards in Healthcare*. HMSO, London.

Department of Health (1994). *The Evolution of Clinical Audit*. HMSO, London.

NHSE (1995). *The New Health Authorities and the Clinical Audit Initiative: Outline of Planned Monitoring Arrangements*. EL(95)103, 4 October. NHSE, Leeds.

NHSE (1996). *Promoting Clinical Effectiveness – A Framework for Action In and Through the NHS*. Crown Copyright. NHSE, Leeds.

2
Evolution of clinical audit

Introduction

The previous chapter outlined the origins and introduction of clinical audit as a mechanism for setting and monitoring standards of clinical practice with a view to improving the quality of healthcare provision in the UK. During the first 5 years, vast resources were invested in education, training and provision of practical support for clinicians in their clinical audit endeavours. Increasing sophistication and effectiveness of clinical audit programmes within provider units have added to the exponential growth of the national knowledge base which, in turn, has enabled the clinical audit process to evolve rapidly and to expand its usefulness, particularly in the areas of guideline development and as a tool to promote clinical effectiveness. The current chapter describes some of the ways in which clinical audit has evolved over recent years and gives an overview of national initiatives in audit, both generally and pertaining to physiotherapy.

National audit projects

Following the changes to funding arrangements for clinical audit at purchaser and provider level as outlined in the previous chapter, the NHS Executive of the Department of Health (NHSE) has continued to support national clinical audit projects from the centrally-held fund.

Information gathered through audit of practice on a nationwide basis provides an overview of the effectiveness of interventions that can help inform development of clinical guidelines based on research evidence. In addition, the NHSE has suggested that reliable clinical guidelines must be amenable to monitoring through the clinical audit process (NHSE, 1996a).

Role of colleges and professional bodies

Since 1989, a proportion of the funding held centrally for medical and clinical audit has been used to support the clinical audit initiatives of, initially, the medical royal colleges and their faculties (Amess *et al.*, 1995) and, latterly, the clinical audit work of the non-medical colleges and professional bodies. The colleges and professional bodies were invited to bid against centrally-held funds for monies which would enable them to set up infrastructures for clinical audit and to employ national advisers to support the audit activities of their members.

In March 1994, the Chartered Society of Physiotherapy (CSP) made a successful bid for central funding to support the establishment of a clinical audit base within the Society's headquarters and, in September 1994, a clinical audit development officer was appointed to develop clinical audit focused upon the work of chartered physiotherapists. A key objective was to carry out a mapping exercise to determine levels of involvement and progress in clinical audit throughout the profession nationally, and to determine the levels of support required for physiotherapy audit initiatives at local level (Hartigan, 1994). The CSP Clinical Audit Development Group was formed in 1995, comprising officers from the Professional Affairs Department and physiotherapists with clinical audit expertise across the UK. Later renamed the Clinical Effectiveness Development Group, a major role of the group remains the support and development of clinical audit within the profession. Ongoing advice on clinical audit initiatives in physiotherapy can be obtained by contacting the Professional Affairs Department at the CSP.

The Department of Health has commissioned the establishment of a national clinical audit and dissemination centre, the National Centre for Clinical Audit (NCCA), 'to ensure that existing and future projects whether national or local are fully informed about similar or related projects' (NCCA, 1996). The NCCA is a partnership of healthcare organizations, led jointly by the British Medical Association (BMA) and the Royal College of Nursing, to facilitate best clinical audit practice on a national basis. The CSP was invited to join the partnership in the summer of 1995, and individual physiotherapists can make use of the vast clinical audit resources offered by the NCCA by contacting the Professional Affairs Department at the CSP in the first instance.

Development of clinical audit in physiotherapy

The different approaches to clinical audit adopted by different professions were discussed briefly in the previous chapter and it was mentioned that early audits in the non-medical clinical professions have tended to concentrate mostly on organizational issues and non-clinical quality standards. Many physiotherapists have also been involved in documentation audit and this is generally regarded as a valid starting point (audits of documentation and record keeping are generally very effective – with vast improvements tending to occur almost immediately the audit begins!).

A report published by CASPE Research (Ramsey *et al.*, 1994) confirmed that, while medical audit programmes had been established in virtually all provider units in England, progress towards multiprofessional clinical audit had been slow and there had been difficulty in ensuring equity in the allocation of audit funding to all healthcare professions. In addition, the mapping exercise carried out by the CSP in 1994/95 suggested that physiotherapists were under-represented in clinical audit at corporate level locally and that only a small number received administrative/computer support for their clinical audit activities from local clinical audit departments.

The changes in funding for audit, as outlined above, highlight a greater need for physiotherapists to move on from documentation and organizational audit activity (although these activities will continue to remain important as part of the contracted service provision) and to concentrate more on addressing discrete aspects of physiotherapeutic practice in a critical manner. It is the effectiveness of physiotherapeutic interventions, both clinically and financially, which will be of greatest interest to health authorities and GP fundholders, and clinical audit programmes must be developed which will demonstrate the effectiveness of physiotherapy treatment in healthcare. As health authorities have been formally charged with promoting participation in clinical audit by *all* healthcare professionals, as outlined above, it is likely that support for audit initiatives in physiotherapy at local level will be easier to obtain in the future. In addition, NHS trusts have been encouraged by the NHSE to consider provision of 'protected time', including clinical cover, to enable clinicians to make use of the educational resources available and to keep up to date on clinical audit issues (NHSE, 1996b).

Evolution of clinical audit as a tool to promote improvement of clinical effectiveness

Throughout the period since 1989, there has been a vast expenditure, from the national NHS budget allocation, on the introduction, development and evolution of clinical audit as a process of critically examining clinical practice against associated resources and seeking to improve the effectiveness of patient care on the basis of audit results.

At its most basic level, clinical audit is a professionally-led initiative which seeks to improve the effectiveness of patient care within local provider units by the setting and monitoring of standards for clinical practice. However, as the process of clinical audit has become embedded into the NHS culture and has been accepted as an essential part of clinical practice in all healthcare professions, new gains from clinical audit have been identified, in particular its important roles in clinical guideline development and promoting the improvement of clinical effectiveness.

Clinical audit is a powerful tool with much scope to evolve further. The NHSE is committed to sustaining ongoing efforts to ensure that clinical audit achieves its full potential, illustrated by the funding of a National Centre for Clinical Audit (NCCA) to promote best practice gained from local initiatives and experiences in multiprofessional audit, and also by publishing guidance urging health authorities and NHS trusts to work together to agree effective local audit programmes which are essential to the success and further development of the tool (NHSE, 1996b).

Similarly, the NHSE approach to the production of clinical guidelines, whether national or local, includes the specific requirement that guidelines should be amenable to clinical audit so that they can be monitored with a view to improving clinical effectiveness. Increasingly, programmes of clinical audit agreed between health authorities and trusts are including requirements for guidelines to be developed and monitored through audit (NHSE, 1996b).

Everyone working professionally within the NHS has a role to play in seeking evidence as to what constitutes clinical effectiveness in healthcare. Reviewing professional practice locally, through the process of clinical audit, together with analysis of the findings and the introduction of change to improve patient care, is the start-point in the promotion of improved clinical effectiveness.

Continuing importance of clinical audit

The continuing importance of the development of clinical audit in physiotherapy, and throughout healthcare, can be summarized as follows.

Clinical audit is integral to the contracting process between purchasers and providers of healthcare, and the placing of contracts for physiotherapy services will increasingly depend upon evidence of the effectiveness of physiotherapeutic interventions as demonstrated by reliable clinical auditing.

Clinical audit is a key component in the development and implementation of strategies to improve the effectiveness of clinical care in the UK.

In line with guidance from the NHSE, the purchasers of healthcare services have an expectation that clinical audit will demonstrate both the clinical effectiveness and cost effectiveness of the services which they are purchasing on behalf of patients.

Doctors are increasingly required to provide evidence, through the use of reliable outcome measurement in medical audit, that a medical/surgical intervention represents the best use of resources and results in the best possible outcome for a particular patient group; as audit contracts become more sophisticated, the onus upon other professions to develop, through the clinical audit process, measurable standards which reflect the effectiveness of their own clinical interventions will increase. It is not an oversimplification to state that clinical audit is about demonstrating achievement of the best possible outcome for the patient, within the resources available.

There will be increasing reference to clinical audit in nursing and paramedical job descriptions and interviews, because of market forces and the need for continued professional development; it is feasible that the requirement to perform clinical audit could be incorporated into the future employment contracts of all healthcare professionals.

Continued professional development in physiotherapy remains as important as ever in the new, primary-led NHS, if not more so given the emergence of professions which will increasingly compete for healthcare contracts, or aspects of service provision, in areas of practice traditionally exclusive to physiotherapy, i.e. chiropractic and osteopathy, generic health workers, and the exponential growth and increasing recognition of alternative therapies in general. In this scenario, clinical audit becomes the tool by which to highlight the unique skills of the physiotherapy profession and to provide evidence to the purchasers of healthcare that physiotherapy is a clinically valuable and cost-effective service that provides high quality care to NHS consumers and their agents, and benefits the population at large.

References

Amess M., Walshe K., Shaw C., Coles J. (1995). *The Audit Activities of the Medical Royal Colleges and Their Faculties in England*. CASPE Research, London.

Hartigan G. (1994). Demystifying clinical audit. *Physiotherapy*, **80**, 863–868.

NCCA (1996). NCCA *Criteria for Clinical Audit*. National Centre for Clinical Audit, Tavistock Square, London.

NHSE (1996a). *Clinical Guidelines – Using Clinical Guidelines to Improve Patient Care Within the NHS*. Crown Copyright. NHSE, Leeds.

NHSE (1996b). *Promoting Clinical Effectiveness – A Framework for Action In and Through the NHS*. Crown Copyright. NHSE, Leeds.

Ramsey M., Walshe K., Bennett J., Coles J. (1994). *The Development of Audit – Findings of a National Survey of Healthcare Provider Units in England*. CASPE Research, London.

3
Defining clinical audit

Clinical audit likened to a Swiss army knife – a multi-faceted tool

We have seen previously that, from its early origins as a means of setting standards for and monitoring the quality of healthcare interventions provided by clinicians, the clinical audit process has evolved and expanded in its usefulness, particularly in the areas of clinical guideline development (NHSE, 1996a) and the promotion of clinical effectiveness. Clinical audit maintains close links with research, supports the development of evidence-based healthcare provision and, increasingly, is expected to inform the contracting process between health authorities and NHS trusts by integrating information on cost and clinical effectiveness and demonstrating local patterns of care (NHSE, 1996b). Clinical audit is first and foremost a tool for clinicians; Figure 3.1 illustrates some of the many areas where the tool is valuable and can be usefully employed.

Practical definitions

Clinical audit was defined by the Department of Health (1994) as the 'systematic, critical analysis of the procedures used for diagnosis, care and treatment, examining how associated resources are used, and investigating the effect that care has on the outcome and quality of life for the patient'.

It has been stated that the official definition was left intentionally vague and deliberately non-prescriptive so that physiotherapists, and other clinicians, might feel free to choose methods and topics for audit which, professionally, they deemed most appropriate, and to audit areas and aspects of care which were judged to be of priority to the individual professions involved.

The ultimate aim of clinical audit in all professions is the improvement of patient care; it is important that it should not be viewed as a management 'weapon' to justify unwelcome service cuts, but as a self-regulatory tool to be used confidently by physiotherapists, to demonstrate improvements in their clinical practice, to enhance clinical education and to further the development of the physiotherapy profession within the wider NHS.

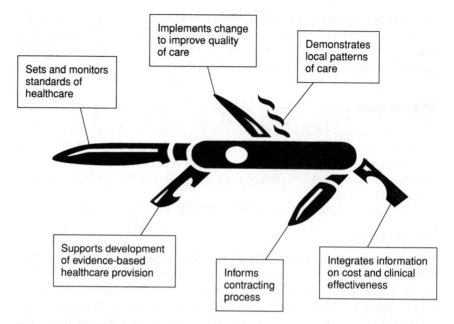

Sets and monitors standards of healthcare

Implements change to improve quality of care

Demonstrates local patterns of care

Supports development of evidence-based healthcare provision

Informs contracting process

Integrates information on cost and clinical effectiveness

Figure 3.1 Clinical audit – a multi-faceted tool

However, some clinicians have remained unhappy with both the vagueness and the 'jargonese' inherent in the official definition and many simpler definitions have been recorded. The most concise is the definition provided by Professor John Gabbay (South and West Regional Health Authority Regional Audit Conference, Poole, 1993): '*Audit is the study of actual practice versus the concept of good practice*'.

This is a very succinct and plain English definition of clinical audit, but even this appears to allude to the idea of standards being imposed upon local physiotherapists by external agencies, i.e. *whose* 'concept of good practice'? In this regard, the definition of the Department of Health is more helpful with its instruction to examine 'the use of associated resources' (Department of Health, 1994), which at least introduces the concept of local ownership and allows one to regard clinical audit as a method of comparing what actually happens in a local unit with the best that could possibly happen, taking local resource limitations into account.

Combining the best of both descriptions allows for a further simplification of the definition of audit and the authors suggest the following:

> Clinical audit is the means of demonstrating that you are providing the most effective clinical service possible within the resources at your disposal.

This latter definition removes all suspicion that clinical audit is a demand on physiotherapists in local units to adhere to standards which have been set externally, and reinforces the concept of local ownership which is essential if clinical audit is to be meaningful and to result in improvements in the quality of patient care.

There is a common misunderstanding among many healthcare professionals that the term 'clinical audit' always refers to multiprofessional team activity, but this is not the case and further definitions given below may help clarify the situation.

Medical audit

Medical audit currently means any audit done by doctors relating to medical care only. For example, percentage of patients up to date with vaccinations, appropriateness of drug prescribing, etc. (The authors hope that this will come to be referred to under the umbrella term 'clinical audit' in the future.)

Clinical audit

Clinical audit refers to audit of any other area, or areas, of clinical practice by any other clinical profession, or professions (including the medical profession in the case of multiprofessional clinical audit). Therefore, in physiotherapy, clinical audit may be uniprofessional (pertaining just to physiotherapy services provided) or multiprofessional (pertaining to the physiotherapist's role in the multiprofessional team).

It is also worth mentioning here that the correct adjective to describe a team of clinicians from different professions is 'multiprofessional' and pointing out that 'multidisciplinary' does not necessarily denote different professions but can also refer to different disciplines within the field of medicine (such as anaesthetics, neurology, radiology, etc. – i.e. medical audit only).

Audit cycle

As demonstrated above, there are many interpretations of the definition of clinical audit, none of which is particularly helpful in indicating what is required in practical terms. Physiotherapists, and other clinicians, have always sought ways of improving patient care; clinical audit is merely a method of improving patient care on a systematic basis.

Clinical audit involves more than just counting events, presenting clinical cases or discussing the various interventions available; clinical audit represents a cycle of activities which, if followed in sequence, should result in the required improvement. This is known as the audit cycle and has been depicted in a variety of published illustrations – in some, it is represented as a complicated flow-chart incorporating all eventualities, in others as a spiral to denote the requirement for systematic audit activity. Figure 3.2 offers a simplified version, the lower section of which (linked by heavy arrows) depicts the major stages of the audit cycle which can be applied to any clinical situation, whilst the upper section (linked by broken-line arrows) illustrates the more complex relationships and roles of clinical audit in the broader initiative of promoting clinical effectiveness.

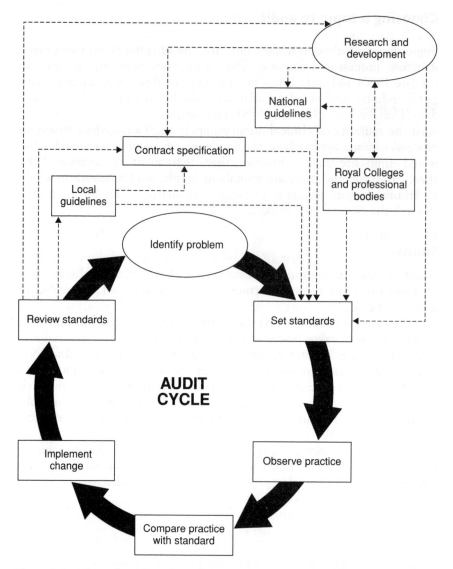

Figure 3.2   The audit cycle and its role in the national clinical effectiveness strategy

Gaining experience in applying the basic audit cycle to discrete aspects of clinical care locally is the first step towards understanding how the process of clinical audit fits into the national clinical effectiveness strategy. It is important to note that, although many external factors and agencies may inform or impact upon the local standard-setting process, the responsibility for identifying and solving problems within a service remains a uniquely local one.

Choosing a topic to audit

Topics for clinical audit usually fall into one of three broad categories – structure, process and outcome. These categories were first described in the late 1950s and early 1960s in relation to quality assurance initiatives in US industry, and were later adapted to the healthcare field by Donabedian (Donabedian, 1966 and 1988). The authors of this book, in common with the majority of clinical auditors, apply the Donabedian structure/process/outcome approach to the implementation of clinical audit, but would emphasize that, in practice, there is frequent overlapping of the three categories and these are formalized simply as a framework in which to ensure that *all* elements of healthcare delivery can be monitored through the clinical audit process.

Structure

Audit of structure is primarily concerned with organizational issues, i.e. anything to do with the actual structure of the organization responsible for delivery of care.

A structure audit might investigate the quality of the environment in which treatment takes place, and it is easy to visualize the internal and external buildings as forming part of the structure of an organization.

However, an audit of waiting times for appointments would also be a structure audit, as the appointments system is part of the way in which an organization structures its services. Another example would be an audit of waiting times in clinic, usually dependent upon availability of staff – staffing levels are also part of the structure of an organization.

Structure audit more properly comes under the heading of organizational audit rather than clinical audit (although there is obviously an overlap) and it is in this area that physiotherapists have tended to concentrate their audit activity in the past.

Process

Audit of process is concerned with all aspects of the actual processing of the patient through the episode of healthcare, from initial assessment through discharge to end of follow-up.

An audit of process could cover areas such as the time it takes for letters or summaries to reach the referring agency, as communication with the referrer is an integral clinical responsibility in the process of delivering healthcare. Audit of physiotherapy documentation is also a process audit, as recording of the interventions provided is part of the clinical process of delivering care.

More often, audit of process considers the actual physiotherapeutic intervention which the patient receives (i.e. the 'hands on' aspect of physiotherapy practice).

A process audit could look at the appropriateness of a variety of physiotherapeutic interventions for a particular client group, based on published standards or research evidence as to which interventions have been proven to be most effective and cost effective.

Audit of process could also highlight the value of a multiprofessional approach to patient care. A multiprofessional process audit might result in the use of multiprofessional clinical records or anticipated recovery pathways, of collaborative goal setting (with each profession contributing in its particular area of expertise), or discharge planning by a multiprofessional team. Discharge planning is likely to cross the primary/secondary interface and require integrated involvement from GPs and other clinicians in the community.

Generally speaking, an integrated, multiprofessional approach to both clinical practice and clinical audit results in greater efficiency all round and increased patient satisfaction.

Outcome

All process audits require some form of outcome measurement and it is questionable whether audit of outcome is pertinent in its own right, without concurrently considering the organizational structure and/or clinical process upon which any outcome depends (Crombie et al., 1993; Kogan et al., 1995). An exception is the area of patient satisfaction which, it should be noted, is strictly a measurement of outcome of intervention in clinical audit, despite its obvious subjectivity.

In most other areas of physiotherapeutic practice, any improvements in the outcome of healthcare delivery for patients can inevitably be achieved only by change(s) to the organizational structure or the contributory clinical process, or both.

However, audit of outcome will be required increasingly by purchasers seeking evidence of the quality of services purchased, and by clinicians both in the development of clinical guidelines and in pursuit of clinical and cost effectiveness.

Measuring the precise outcome of a specific intervention by a clinician of any profession is fraught with difficulties and often subject to influence by outside factors, such as natural recovery, home environment, social class, patient compliance, etc. Despite ,this, audit of outcome is not necessarily difficult, nor does it always involve the use of complicated outcome measurement tools. Clinical audit identifies local trends and patterns, and it may be possible to set standards for both process and outcome (or structure and outcome) using physiotherapeutic judgement in the context of the patterns which emerge.

For many local audits, patterns of shorter duration of admission because of physiotherapeutic intervention, increased functional mobility, earlier return to work through improved patient education or compliance, or earlier discharge from follow-up, will suffice.

However, when unequivocal evidence of health outcome attributable to physiotherapy intervention is needed (e.g. in the development of clinical guidelines), there are a number of sophisticated outcome measurement tools available. The best of these will have been validated through previous audit or research projects, and many can be easily adapted for differing clinical situations. Outcome measurement and outcome audit are considered in detail in Chapters 11 and 12 respectively.

References

Crombie I.K., Davies H.T.O., Abraham S.C.S., Florey C. du V. (1993). *The Audit Handbook: Improving Health Care Through Clinical Audit*. John Wiley and Sons, Chichester.

Department of Health (1994). *The Evolution of Clinical Audit*. HMSO, London.

Donabedian A. (1966). *Evaluating the Quality of Medical Care*. Millbank Memorial Federation of Quality, USA. Part 3, pp. 166–203.

Donabedian A. (1988). The quality of care: how can it be assessed? *Journal of the American Medical Association*, **260**, 1743–1748.

Kogan M., Redfern S., with Kober A., Norman I., Packwood T., Robinson S. (1995). *Making Use of Clinical Audit*. Open University Press, Milton Keynes.

NHSE (1996a). *Clinical Guidelines – Using Clinical Guidelines to Improve Patient Care Within the NHS*. Crown Copyright. NHSE, Leeds.

NHSE (1996b). *Promoting Clinical Effectiveness – A Framework for Action In and Through the NHS*. Crown Copyright. NHSE, Leeds.

4

Basic requirements for clinical audit in physiotherapy

Obtaining support for physiotherapy audit within NHS provider units

A clinical audit project on a single topic usually requires a couple of meetings of all members of staff who will be involved in the audit, to discuss the topic to be audited and to agree the clinical standards against which practice is to be measured. It often also involves designing forms, data collection sheets and questionnaires, input and analysis of data collected and production of reports—all of which would rightly be regarded as tedious and time-consuming chores for practising physiotherapists with busy clinical workloads. Some physiotherapists may have no prior experience with database and spreadsheet software packages and may feel reluctant to get involved in any clinical audit project because of the vast amount of administration which they may perceive will be required of them.

It is therefore important to stress that it is *not* the responsibility of any physiotherapist to sit up until midnight using a personal computer at home, or work through lunch breaks, or work late, dealing with the administrative aspects of clinical audit.

Every acute provider unit/trust should now have a clinical audit committee (as opposed to a medical audit committee) and all professions should be represented thereon. It is not unusual for one member of the paramedical professions to represent up to two others, but the scenario of a clinician of one profession representing nine other professions, both paramedical and non-paramedical, should no longer exist. It is the collective responsibility of the clinical audit committee to ensure that adequate support is provided for clinical audit initiatives in all professions.

Importantly, every acute provider unit/trust should have a corporate clinical audit department which employs staff for the sole purpose of providing clerical/secretarial/computer support for audit initiatives in all clinical professions. Similar arrangements exist in community trusts and via the Multiprofessional Audit Advisory Groups (MAAGs) in the community setting.

Corporate clinical audit departments offer a wide range of support services for clinical audit activity, although these vary from hospital to hospital and depend largely upon the staffing levels of the audit department itself. Some of the bigger teaching hospitals provide a designated audit assistant for physiotherapy audit to advise on design of projects and to help with collection, analysis and reporting of data. In other units, audit assistants are shared between services and may support a number of simultaneous projects at different stages of the audit cycle. In yet other hospitals, clinicians apply formally to the clinical audit committee for support with audit initiatives and each project is judged upon its merits.

If physiotherapists are unaware of the availability of these facilities or how to harness them for audit activity, they should make enquiries within their directorates or via their service managers, or with their representative on the clinical audit committee. In many cases, a simple telephone call to the clinical audit co-ordinator/facilitator should prove useful. The input to clinical audit by physiotherapists should never involve more than contributing to the setting of clinical standards, perhaps ticking boxes on data sheets when writing up the clinical record (often the most efficient way to collect concurrent data), adhering to the standards in the clinical setting, and acting upon the results of audit activity to implement change and improve the quality of care.

Organizing a programme of clinical audit activity

It is impossible for every aspect of care to be audited at once but it is feasible to have several projects underway at different stages of the audit cycle at any one time. Instituting regular audit meetings (perhaps designating one in-service meeting of the physiotherapy department on a regular basis as an official audit meeting), whereby updates on all projects can be given to the entire service, helps to maintain momentum and engender fresh interest. Meaningful audits should contribute to in-service training and clinical education by encouraging discussion about the priority of audit topics and the findings of literature reviews, and by the sharing of clinical information throughout a physiotherapy service.

An example of a rolling clinical audit programme for a physiotherapy service, combining community services and acute hospital provision within a single NHS trust, for one financial year, is illustrated at Table 4.1.

Setting standards for clinical audit

If the aims of clinical audit are to demonstrate the best possible local practice and result in an improvement in the quality of patient care, then achievement of these aims must depend upon the existence of local

Table 4.1 Rolling programme of physiotherapy clinical audit activity

	Community service	Acute hospital provision
April	Discharge letters **(Process)**	Waiting times in clinic **(Structure)**
May		Pre-operative physiotherapy assessment of total knee replacements **(Process and outcome)**
June	Audit of documentation **(Process)**	↑
July		
August		↕
September	Waiting list for appointments **(Structure)**	
October		↓
November	Treatment of medical chests **(Process and outcome)**	
December	↑	
January		Audit of documentation **(Process)**
February	↕	
March	↓	Outpatient satisfaction survey **(Outcome)**

standards for best possible practice, against which actual practice can be measured.

It is solely for physiotherapists to decide and agree what the local standard should be for any particular aspect of physiotherapy practice. Before a decision is reached, it is important to review the clinical literature to ascertain what is universally accepted as best practice, and to review any relevant guidelines from the CSP, followed by a period of discussion as to how these 'paper' standards can be adapted to clinical practice in the local setting. For example, in June 1993, the CSP published its second edition of *Standards of Physiotherapy Practice* (Chartered Society of Physiotherapy, 1993) which provides broad-based guidance for general physiotherapeutic practice and could be expanded upon and incorporated into local clinical audit standards. In addition, many physiotherapy clinical interest groups have produced standards or guidelines for specialist areas of clinical practice. Most standards and guidelines are written with a view to regular revision. Contact the appropriate clinical interest group and the CSP for the latest physiotherapy updates in specific areas of practice.

Local clinical audit standards are then set by consensus of the physiotherapists involved, who will endeavour to adhere to them in practice. Many methods exist for auditing clinical practice against agreed standards and these are considered in detail in the next chapter.

Commitment to change

The overriding objective of clinical audit is to improve patient care. If a physiotherapy standard has been set within a local unit as to what constitutes optimal care in that unit, and audit of actual practice reveals that the standard is not being met, there must be a commitment on the part of the auditing physiotherapists to change either the practice or the standard; there is no point in any audit taking place without a commitment to change.

It should be noted, however, that a very low percentage achievement may indicate that the original standard was set too high and may need to be reconsidered; it could be that certain factors were overlooked when the standard was set, or that a subgroup of patients should have been excluded from the sample because of unique or intractable problems. Similarly, a 100% achievement probably means that the standard was set too low. As experience in clinical audit increases, it becomes easier to define clinical standards with greater accuracy and to gain insight into obvious exclusions.

Clinical audit should be viewed as part of continuous quality improvement in clinical practice. If an audit demonstrates that agreed standards are not being achieved and that changes to local practice are necessary, it is important to review practice again to ensure that any relevant changes have been implemented and that implementation has indeed resulted in the agreed standards being achieved. In most cases, awareness of the under-achievement of the standard and a concerted effort to change a particular aspect of clinical practice will result in the standard being achieved at a second audit. Re-auditing to ensure that change has been implemented is known as 'closing the audit loop'.

Reluctance by clinicians to accept the changes indicated by audit was cited as a major constraint on progress with clinical audit in a 1995 survey of audit in the therapy professions (Redfern et al., 1995). This highlights the importance of involving all clinicians from the outset in any audit which may impact upon their practice.

Role of physiotherapy manager in clinical audit

A fundamental principle of the Department of Health's policy statement on clinical audit was that it should involve managers as well as clinicians (Department of Health, 1994).

It has been stated previously that clinical audit is a professionally led and educationally based activity and a self-regulatory tool with which clinicians can review their practice, set clinical standards and implement changes to improve the quality of patient care. There are no grounds for regarding clinical audit as a 'weapon' wielded by management to impose unwelcome changes on physiotherapeutic practice. However, because it is managers who have overall responsibility for the quality of care delivered, they need to be aware of, involved in and committed to the clinical audit activity which is undertaken within their departments. It is managers in NHS provider units who will agree contracts for both clinical service delivery and clinical audit programmes with purchasing health authorities, and they need to be fully informed of local audit activity in order to optimize their participation in contract negotiations.

In its guidance on promoting clinical effectiveness, the NHSE stated that the informed participation of managers is essential to the success and further development of clinical audit, and emphasized that managers need to agree local programmes of audit activity with both clinicians and purchasers (NHSE, 1996). Managers are further urged to provide financial resources to enable clinicians to remain up to date individually with clinical audit issues, and support for library services, training events and clinical cover.

Locally, managers need to be involved in clinical audit for the simple reason that audit activity may reveal deficiencies in the running of the organization as well as highlighting areas where clinical practice might be improved and, in this situation, active involvement by managers at the outset is more likely to result in a commitment to implement organizational change. Delivery of quality care is dependent upon the members of the healthcare team working together, both interprofessionally and in association with their managers, to ensure that the best possible service is provided.

Because of the initial funding mechanism for clinical audit, examined earlier, it has not been possible for many physiotherapists to be at the forefront of clinical audit activity, and uncertainty and confusion continue to exist in some areas, particularly concerning the rationale behind clinical audit and its benefits for the physiotherapy profession. Physiotherapy managers have a vital role to play in this regard by encouraging their staff to build up knowledge and confidence in practical clinical audit activity, and by providing support for training initiatives wherever possible (Hartigan, 1994).

Perhaps the most important contribution of a physiotherapy manager is to provide a non-threatening environment where physiotherapists can examine aspects of clinical care on a systematic basis. Gaining a comprehensive understanding of the aims and benefits of clinical audit in physiotherapy, through regular participation on a uniprofessional basis and with the support of a sympathetic manager, will be the key to greater involvement in multiprofessional clinical audit activity in line with national strategy.

As contracts for clinical audit become more sophisticated, the management contribution will need to be further expanded so that the generation of health outcome data can be incorporated into strategic management planning and contract negotiation. Managers should ensure that appropriate structures are in place to support systematic clinical audit activity within a service, and that staff are adequately educated in the importance and impact of clinical audit on delivery of healthcare services.

References

Chartered Society of Physiotherapy (1993). *Standards of Physiotherapy Practice*, 2nd edn. 14 Bedford Row, London WC1R 4ED.

Department of Health (1994). *The Evolution of Clinical Audit*. HMSO, London.

Hartigan G. (1994). The role of the manager in clinical audit. *Journal of the Association of Chartered Physiotherapists in Management*, Winter.

NHSE (1996). *Promoting Clinical Effectiveness – A Framework for Action In and Through the NHS*. Crown Copyright. NHSE, Leeds.

Redfern S., Kogan M., Kober A., Norman I., Robinson S., Packwood T. (1995). *Clinical Audit in Four Health Professions*. Report to the Department of Health, Centre for the Evaluation of Public Policy and Practice, Uxbridge and London: Brunel University and Nursing Research Unit, King's College, London University.

5
Clinical audit methods

Clinical audit methods explained

There are many methods, and surprisingly few rules governing which to select, for conducting clinical audit activity within a service. For the audit beginner, this can be bewildering, frustrating and ultimately off-putting (Hartigan, 1995). However, deciding which clinical audit method to use is solely dependent upon the aims of the audit, the type and quantity of audit data to be collected, and the hoped-for results of the exercise (Joint Centre for Education in Medicine, 1992). For example, a straightforward documentation audit is unlikely to produce the data required to compare outcomes of intervention for a particular client group—an additional means of collecting data would be required, concentrating on outcome information. Likewise, a criterion-based audit would not produce information on patient satisfaction unless a supplementary questionnaire was designed at the outset. The main factors to be considered are ease and completeness of data collection, and achievement of the initial aims of the audit.

The most common methods used in clinical audit are summarized below, including a brief description in simple language of what is involved for each method at a practical level (Hartigan, 1995; reproduced with permission).

I. Documentation or note-keeping audit

There are few, if any, physiotherapists who have not been involved in some kind of documentation audit in which a standard is set, describing the minimum information which the clinical record should contain and the expected degree of clarity and legibility, and the case notes then examined to measure adherence to the standard.

Although audit of documentation may seem unexciting from a clinical viewpoint, it can be regarded as clinical audit in its truest sense and it is generally regarded as a valid starting point for clinical audit activity.

Physiotherapists have a legal, professional duty to maintain clear, accurate, up to date and legible records of the clinical treatments given, so an audit of documentation addresses an important area of clinical and professional practice. (It is also one of the few areas of clinical audit where change takes place well in advance of completion of the audit, with the standard of documentation improving almost immediately by virtue of the knowledge that record-keeping is being monitored!)

2. Case note analysis

Case note analysis involves the random selection of a small number of case notes, usually of patients with the same diagnosis, which are then reviewed on the basis of the treatments given. The findings may be presented to an in-service meeting of the local physiotherapy group to engender discussion on the methods of treatment available for that diagnosis.

Although this method contributes to the educational aspect of the clinical audit process, it does not represent a complete audit because it does not usually result in a change of clinical practice. However, it may throw up ideas for topics of audit by other methods or play a part in standard setting in areas such as the appropriateness of the methods of treatment used.

3. Criterion-based audit

This method of audit is probably used most commonly throughout health-care and consists of comparing explicit, measurable criteria or specific standards, for a particular aspect of care, with the care that is actually provided in the clinical setting. The 'criteria' are merely a list of things which should happen if the standard has been achieved, set out on a data collection sheet, which can then be checked against the information in the clinical records. Both the standards and the criteria are agreed by physiotherapists at the outset of the audit.

For example, a physiotherapy standard may state that quads power and range of movement should be measured and recorded for all patients with a particular diagnosis. The criteria for the audit in this case would read:

Quads power recorded?   YES/NO
Range of movement recorded?   YES/NO

An advantage of criterion-based audit is that, once standards and explicit criteria have been agreed by physiotherapists, the actual trawl through the patients' records (the audit) can be performed by audit department staff or any available support staff (i.e. assistants, departmental secretaries, etc.), thus saving valuable clinical time, although the physiotherapists would be required to review and disseminate the results of each audit so that improvements could be made in the case of clinical deficiency.

4. Adverse occurrence screening

Adverse occurrence screening is not a complete method of audit and is more likely to be used in nursing or medical audit rather than an audit of physiotherapeutic practice.

It usually takes place in the acute hospital setting when events occur that are not commonly associated with either the disease process or any of the treatments given, e.g. falls on a ward, unplanned returns to the operating theatre, infection from blood transfusion.

Screening of such adverse events on a systematic basis is a method of identifying trends and patterns; once a pattern emerges, the reasons for the problem (which may be a management problem or a clinical problem) can be investigated, standards developed and changes in practice implemented. In the case of clinical deficiency, criterion-based audit would usually follow to ensure that the new standards were being met.

5. Patient survey

Patient surveys are a valuable means of receiving feedback from the users of clinical services and involve the use of a simple questionnaire to determine whether certain pre-set standards have been met.

Questions should be unambiguous and formulated in plain language to which the answer can be a simple.'yes' or 'no'. For example, if a physiotherapy outpatient standard states that an information leaflet should be given to all patients at the first appointment, the question would ask:

Did you receive an information leaflet at your first outpatient appointment?

This may seem glaringly obvious in principle but, in practice, it is all too easy to ask a question which takes certain information for granted, or a question that is difficult to answer simply, as in the following two examples:

Were you satisfied with the physiotherapist's explanation of your treatment?
(Presupposes that an explanation of some kind was received – a negative answer would be assumed to refer to the satisfaction aspect only.)

Was the physiotherapy waiting area clean and comfortable?
(May have been one but not the other.)

Because questionnaires address specific areas within an episode of care, it is fairly straightforward to implement changes on the basis of results. A repeat audit using the same questionnaire after a period of time would indicate whether improvement had been achieved, thereby closing the audit loop.

6. Peer review

The term 'peer review', in its truest sense, means the process by which the work of an individual is reviewed by a peer of the individual, with 'peer' meaning one who is equal clinically, in grade, qualification, expertise, etc.

In the early days of medical audit, it was suggested that all completed audits should be subject to peer review, i.e. that an audit performed by one group of doctors should be evaluated by another group of doctors from the same medical specialty, with comparable clinical skills and expertise, but perhaps from another unit. It is hardly surprising that, in practice, this rarely happened, both because of the time factor involved in auditing the same data twice and also because of the element of competitiveness which such a practice introduces.

A peer review audit in physiotherapy might involve summarizing a patient assessment from the case notes of an unidentified physiotherapist and asking another (similarly unidentified) physiotherapist of a similar grade and experience to suggest a management and treatment plan on the basis of the information given; differences in clinical opinion could be discussed by a meeting of the physiotherapy group, taking scrupulous care not to identify any of the physiotherapists involved.

As in case note analysis, this audit method contributes to clinical education but does not represent true audit, since it is rarely performed on a systematic basis and does not necessarily result in change of practice or improvement of care. Physiotherapy audit by peer review is of limited value; it is invariably viewed as contentious and threatening by the physiotherapists involved, and it introduces an element of competitiveness into a process which requires confidence and consensus if it is to result in meaningful change.

However, every method of audit involves a form of peer review, with peer *groups* of clinicians reviewing methods of treatment and discussing general clinical practice so that standards of patient care can be set by clinical consensus. Reviewing clinical information in a group is generally regarded as less contentious and, on the whole, achieves more positive results.

Clinical audit *versus* research

All the methods suggested above require some kind of measurement of outcome and measuring the specific outcome of a clinical intervention is one of the most difficult aspects of clinical audit. Both outcome measurement and outcome audit in physiotherapy are considered in comprehensive detail in Chapters 11 and 12 of this book, but it is worth mentioning here that it is in this area that the links between clinical audit and research are closest and the distinction between them most blurred.

Clinical audit is not research. Although clear similarities have been drawn between clinical audit and action research (Birkett, 1995), the links and dissimilarities between clinical audit and pure research are more complex.

Research tests new knowledge and methods of treatment, accounting for all possible variables, while clinical audit looks at what actually happens in a specific setting, based on existing validated research (standard setting in clinical audit always begins with a review of the clinical literature), and investigates if there are ways in which patient care can be improved or better use made of resources in that particular setting.

Research is the process which tests non-validated treatments and practices and therefore requires ethical approval and informed patient consent.

Because clinical audit results are always anonymized, because patients are not being entered into a trial whereby they receive untested treatments and are, in fact, receiving standard validated treatments, ethical and informed consent are almost never required before commencing an audit project. (There are rare exceptions to this rule – for example, in the case of a questionnaire survey of carers of patients in a high-mortality diagnostic group, some of whom may have died prior to the survey taking place. Possible sensitivity of an audit topic should be considered before commencement and a common sense approach adopted.)

In clinical audit, the focus is the patient; the focus in research is the method of treatment or knowledge being tested, with the long-term aim of benefiting the future of patient care.

Clinical audit and research can serve to strengthen each other because, if unexpected results occur in an audit, it can provide evidence of the need for research in a particular area; conversely, when research findings have been disseminated, clinical audit becomes the tool by which to monitor their incorporation into routine practice. (All clinical audits should begin with a review of the research literature to assist in establishing standards in the local setting.)

Outcome measurement

A physiotherapy outcome measure is an audit tool that measures the alteration in health or functional status of a patient that is likely to be due to physiotherapy intervention. Outcome measures can be objective (goniometric measurement of range of movement, peak flow, etc.) or subjective from either the physiotherapist's viewpoint (i.e. 'half-range') or from the patient's viewpoint (i.e. 'much better').

It is important that any outcome measure used in physiotherapy audit is accurate, and accuracy is achieved by demonstrating that the particular outcome measure is appropriate (suitable and fitting for what is being measured), reliable (accurate and repeatable when used by other physiotherapists), valid (sound, capable of being justified for use in a particular clinical situation), and responsive (sensitive to slight change).

Full information and many practical examples of physiotherapy outcome measurement are considered in detail in Chapter 11.

References

Birkett M. (1995). Is audit action research? *Physiotherapy*, **81**, 190–194.
Hartigan G. (1995). Choosing a method for clinical audit: the first hurdle. *Physiotherapy*, **81**, 187–188.
Joint Centre for Education in Medicine (1992). *Making Medical Audit Effective*. 13 Millman Street, London WC1N 3EJ.

6
Completing the audit cycle

Acting upon clinical audit results

Clinical audit is not an end in itself, simply a tool which demonstrates commitment to and implementation of a quality, efficient and effective service. It should be emphasized that clinical audit is about making changes, not just collecting data – it is the changes that can be produced in the clinical setting, not the data themselves, which are important (Joint Centre for Education in Medicine, 1992).

Thus, the most important action which physiotherapists can take in the event of clinical audit results demonstrating non-achievement of a standard, which had been agreed to be clinically achievable, is to identify the reasons why the standard was not met and to implement changes to physiotherapeutic practice, thereby ensuring achievement of the standard at re-audit and closing of the audit loop.

The main aim of clinical audit is to improve the quality of patient care; it is therefore important, when selecting a topic for physiotherapy audit, to choose an area of practice where it is commonly felt that there is room for improvement. Although it may be gratifying to see collected and analysed data providing evidence of excellent service, the process of clinical audit is meant to be self-regulatory, not self-congratulatory. It is first and foremost a tool for improving less than optimal service delivery, and also a problem-solving mechanism. In this regard, it is advisable to keep in mind the old maxim, 'if it ain't broke, don't fix it' (Crombie *et al.*, 1993) which, for clinical audit purposes, could be translated into, 'if there is no problem with an aspect of the physiotherapy service, don't audit it'.

Similarly, be sure that the area of practice that is being audited actually *is* physiotherapy practice, over which the physiotherapists have the power, ability and commitment to implement change on the basis of results. It is often easier, more comfortable and less threatening to identify problems in other professional services rather than look too closely at areas of physiotherapy where problems may be suspected. It may be equally tempting to suggest changes to the practice of other professions that might appear obvious to the individual physiotherapist or collective physiotherapy service, but this could never be regarded as clinical audit, which is only concerned with clinicians examining their *own* therapeutic practices.

The reluctance of clinicians to accept the need for changes indicated by clinical audit was described as a constraint on progress with clinical audit in a 1995 survey of audit in the therapy professions (Redfern *et al.*, 1995), and changing practice on the basis of audit results is universally acknowledged as a difficult concept for any healthcare profession. Indeed, it is at this stage of an audit project when commitment and impetus are most likely to falter. This can even result in the abandonment of a project, with attendant disappointment and frustration for the participants, who feel that they have wasted their time collecting the data and may be discouraged from getting involved in audit in the future.

It has been stated previously that there is little point in any audit taking place without a commitment to change on the part of the participating physiotherapists. However, it is worth reiterating that there is sometimes a danger of rushing into an audit on the back of good intentions, without first investigating that the participants are actually empowered to bring about any changes highlighted by the results, nor perhaps ensuring that those whose assistance may be needed to effect change (i.e. managers) have been fully consulted and involved from the outset of the audit.

A well-designed clinical audit project considers not only what the participants want to achieve by their auditing of a specific topic, but also whether the changes are achievable. The audit plan would then include consultation with and commitment from all relevant parties, plus regular review of interim audit results and discussion about how best to implement changes.

A partial audit, to the stage of having analysed the data and agreed on the changes to be implemented, may already have resulted in some improvements in quality – due to awareness of the problem, education through audit and the tendency for practice to begin to change ahead of all the information having been gathered. To optimize the benefits of the audit, it is important to continue with the project and close the audit loop. To facilitate this, a time frame for re-audit, to ensure that suggested changes have been implemented should be written into the initial plan wherever possible.

Disseminating clinical audit results

It is obvious that the results of clinical audit should be shared with all the participating members of the particular physiotherapy group, or multi-professional team, on a regular basis as the audit project progresses, but it is also useful to publicize the anonymized results as widely as possible within the local unit or trust.

In addition, the corporate clinical audit committee should be informed of the audit findings at the end of a project – as well as at the outset – so that purchasers can know that clinical audit activity is going on in that particular area. (Since April 1994, clinical audit committees are required to include a purchasing representative.)

On a wider basis, most non-medical colleges and professional bodies endeavour to keep a database of audits carried out by their members and you may wish to apprise the CSP of your clinical audit activity, for the purposes of information sharing and professional development on a nationwide basis. The National Centre for Clinical Audit (NCCA), of which the CSP is a founder partner, has been commissioned specifically to disseminate information on clinical audit and 'to ensure that existing and future projects whether national or local are fully informed about similar or related projects' (NCCA, 1996).

Finally, publication of physiotherapy audits – either in *Physiotherapy* or in one of the many specialist clinical audit and quality publications – can only add to the development and continued evolution of clinical audit throughout healthcare, and thus enhance education and awareness of the value of clinical audit to the physiotherapy profession.

References

Crombie I.K., Davies H.T.O., Abraham S.C.S., Florey C. du V. (1993). *The Audit Handbook: Improving Health Care Through Clinical Audit*. John Wiley and Sons, Chichester.

Joint Centre for Education in Medicine (1992). *Making Medical Audit Effective*. 13 Millman Street, London WC1N 3EJ.

NCCA (1996). *NCCA Criteria for Clinical Audit*. National Centre for Clinical Audit, Tavistock Square, London.

Redfern S., Kogan M., Kober A., Norman I., Robinson S., Packwood T. (1995). *Clinical Audit in Four Health Professions*. Report to the Department of Health, Centre for the Evaluation of Public Policy and Practice, Uxbridge and London: Brunel University and Nursing Research Unit, King's College, London University.

SECTION 2
INTEGRATING CLINICAL AUDIT INTO PHYSIOTHERAPY PRACTICE

7
From theory into practice

Piecing together the jigsaw

A basic understanding of the principles of clinical audit and a knowledge
of the audit cycle are vital before embarking on an audit project in practice. The first section of this book dealt with the building blocks of clinical audit, what they are, how they have evolved and how they are used in
theory. The second section describes how these building blocks may be put
together to devise specific physiotherapy audits and to link into multiprofessional, interface and inter-agency audits in practice.

As physiotherapists, we strive to give our patients the best possible care,
treatment and advice. 'The best' needs to be identified by experienced clinicians, proven by research and checked by clinical audit, firstly to see that it
is being implemented, and secondly to ascertain whether it is still 'the best'.

Auditing the care element of physiotherapy may involve looking at the
structure and processes whereby a service is offered. Chapter 9 of this book
looks at physiotherapy structure audits and identifies some ways in which
the material and personnel resources available to the service may be
audited to optimize the quality of service provision.

Process audits examine the elements of the processes whereby patients get
into, through and out of the system (Chapter 10). Although this includes
evaluation of the 'hands on' intervention, i.e. treatment and advice, audit
of outcome is considered separately in Chapter 12 in order to address specific outcome audit methodologies in detail. Structure, process and outcome
physiotherapy audits are explained in depth in Chapters 9, 10 and 12.

We have already seen that clinical audit is not research, but it does have
an important role to play in the process of influencing practice and monitoring success (Mann, 1996). Alongside all other healthcare professionals
we strive for clinical effectiveness. Integrating clinical audit into practice
is a systematic method of continual assessment of a physiotherapy service.

Getting physiotherapy audit up and running

The Chartered Society of Physiotherapy (CSP) is committed to clinical
audit. In a position statement on clinical audit, the CSP defined clinical
audit in physiotherapy as:

... the systematic evaluation of service provision. This covers direct and indirect delivery of intervention processes and their subsequent outcomes. Clinical audit data collected provides the meaningful information required to initiate appropriate change, ensure evidence based practice via measurable standards and criteria that will result in the efficient and effective delivery of a quality service for patients and their carers within available resources – monetary, expertise and time related.

(Clinical Audit Development Group, CSP, *Frontline*, July 17 1996.)

As this statement is produced by the professional body, it applies to all chartered physiotherapists whether working in the National Health Service, independent hospitals, private practice or for charitable bodies. Examples of clinical audit may be found in any of these sectors, although all the examples in this book originated in NHS physiotherapy units. The authors are not aware of any published audits undertaken by physiotherapists working in animal therapy, but there is no reason why the audit principles of service evaluation may not be used in this area, and one of the authors outlined ways in which clinical audit theory could be translated to the field of animal therapy for the 1995 Spring Seminar of the Association of Chartered Physiotherapists in Animal Therapy (Hartigan, 1995).

The CSP sees physiotherapy clinical audit as being closely linked with clinical effectiveness, evidence-based practice and physiotherapy education from undergraduate training through to continuing professional development. The CSP recognizes the need for ongoing training in audit and provides training and support from its Professional Affairs Department. However, the time comes when each physiotherapist or department must take the plunge and begin to audit local physiotherapy practice.

In practice, getting physiotherapy audit underway happens in stages. Including the stages described below ensures that the audit cycle is completed. Completion means that the main aim of the audit is fulfilled, i.e. identified shortfalls are attended to and changes implemented. The audit is then repeated to ensure that the new procedures are actually in place (closing the audit loop).

Stages for successful physiotherapy audit in practice

- Managerial commitment to clinical audit
- Departmental commitment to clinical audit
- Address anxieties about audit
- Physiotherapy team brainstorms topics for clinical audit
- Physiotherapy team sets up a programme for addressing each agreed topic
- Physiotherapy team identifies one audit project to start with
- Team draws up an audit protocol and timetable for the first project

- Specify definite aims and objectives
- Consider practicality of the project
- Identify the best practice to use as standards
- Discuss and agree upon the appropriate criteria or outcome measures
- Identify and design the appropriate data collection tool
- Run the audit
- Keep the objectives and timetable under review
- Analyse the results
- Look critically at the results in discussion with the team
- Decide what changes need to be made in order to reach the set standards
- Implement the changes
- Allow a period of time for the changes to take effect
- Re-audit to see if the changes are effective.

Obtaining managerial commitment to clinical audit

As we have seen in the previous section, clinical audit has been around in its present form for several years and is now embedded into contracts. This should ensure a level of managerial commitment to audit because, even if staff are not keen on the concept, a clinical audit element will already have been negotiated and will need to be implemented.

Obtaining departmental commitment to clinical audit

Departmental commitment to clinical audit is another matter. There are many views on the efficacy and need for clinical audit in physiotherapy, some positive, others less so. These reactions to clinical audit are by no means limited to physiotherapists (Crombie *et al.*, 1993). Clinical audit was formally introduced at a time of wide-ranging and rapid changes within the NHS and some of the anxieties about audit relate to the speed of change. Initially, clinical audit was promoted as a form of peer review (Standing Committee on Postgraduate Medical Education, 1989). This was a deliberate attempt to allay anxieties that the non-clinical management within a unit would impose standards on professional autonomy. For some clinicians, however, this had the opposite effect of instilling genuine fear that 'big brother' (in the shape of senior clinicians or non-clinical managers) would begin to criticize individual performance in the form of a witch hunt. In more recent years, the essence of clinical audit has moved towards a team approach to evaluation, with the emphasis on team responsibilities rather than any perceived individual performance. The main aim of clinical audit remains the same: to optimize patient care and service delivery through critical evaluation of the structure, process and outcomes of the service.

Addressing anxieties

Some anxieties are common to physiotherapists undertaking audit.

Anxiety 1: "Audit is time consuming and takes me away from my patients"
This anxiety is well justified as clinical audit can be very time consuming. However, there is no reason why it should impinge intrusively upon patient time.

- Some physiotherapy departments identify a named senior clinician as having audit co-ordinator responsibility as part of his or her managerial duties. Identifying a key person with lead responsibility for an audit within a department channels all enquiries and allows for central management of information rather than a patchy flow. It is vital that all persons involved in the audit should know who the key person is, what his or her responsibilities are and how they can get in touch with him/her.
- Most NHS trusts have a central clinical audit department which can provide the expertise, and often the personnel, to undertake the audit data collection and analysis (see Chapter 4). Funding for this service is negotiated within the service contract.
- In many cases, time spent evaluating service delivery can be recouped in the future by efficiencies made as a result of the audit.

Anxiety 2: "Surely my professional qualifications and experience are assurance enough of the quality of my practice?"
This is true up to a point but, as individual practitioners, we are used to attending courses to update our skills, keeping abreast of the current literature in our particular field of work and setting aims and objectives at annual individual performance reviews. An audit is a review and evaluation of an aspect of service delivery and, although it may well encompass the outcomes of individual therapists' practice, its prime objective is to examine the service as a whole rather than the role of individual members of staff. Just as we need constantly to review personal practice through continuing professional development, so a service needs regular examination to ensure that is functioning as well as possible.

Anxiety 3: "Audit is not only time consuming, it is also a waste of time"
This is a common experience of clinicians who have spent a long time setting up audits which have never been completed, where the recommended changes have never been implemented, or where the results have had little relevance to the service. All of these issues should be addressed at the beginning of the audit.

- In the review of audit activity in the nursing and therapy professions by CASPE Research (Willmott *et al.*, 1995), researchers discovered that only 18% of audits had an identified time span and that only half of audit initiatives had achieved some or all of their aims. It is very common to find the bulk of the enthusiasm for clinical audit occurring in the early planning stages. This enthusiasm wanes over time and, unless there is a key individual working to a protocol, many audits will fail through lack of interest. Clinicians who have experienced this in the past will undoubtedly have major concerns that future audits may follow a similar pattern. However, very many audits have been successful and have changed clinical practice for the better. Examples of these audits can be found in current professional and audit literature, some of which are referred to later in this book.

- The main effect of an uncompleted audit is that no changes can take place. This undermines the whole reason for undertaking the audit in the first place. Before starting an audit ask the following questions:

  Will the staff be *willing* to make any changes found necessary?
  Will the staff be *able* to make any changes found necessary?
  Will recommended changes receive back-up from management?
  Will the necessary resources be available to implement the changes?

  Unless the answers to all these questions are 'yes', the audit may be in vain.

- Audit projects should not only be successfully completed, they should also be worthwhile. Some audits have not delivered usable information as they have asked the wrong questions or collected the wrong data. This may seem an obvious point but it is surprisingly easy to drift from the original audit aim and find out, too late, that the data do not address the initial questions. This can be avoided by writing a protocol that is agreed by all participants, and then keeping closely to it. It may be tempting to 'just gather a little more data while we're about it', but this soon makes a crisp audit unwieldy and dilutes its impact. Taking advice from clinical audit department staff on data collection and the design of data collection tools can also help to keep a project on track.

Anxiety 4: "If our audit results show that we are delivering a poor service, we will lose credibility within the trust and possibly our contract too!"

It is important to emphasize that clinical audit data should be anonymized and that the results of audit are confidential to those undertaking the audit. Clinical audit information may be shared only with the express agreement of all participants. Everyone has the occasional shock when they discover that a service they thought was efficient and effective is in fact a bit of a shambles, leaving much to be desired.

This is the time to use clinical audit to your advantage. You have been pro-active in discovering the shortfall; now is the time to instigate change to address the situation. This puts you very much in control. If you have agreed to share the results of your audit with purchasers of your service, you can emphasize your flexibility and dedication to clinical effectiveness by undertaking the changes indicated by audit. Maintaining a positive attitude is paramount. You may even be able to use clinical audit data to your advantage in negotiating extra funding for staff or equipment. At the end of the day, it is surely better to identify and deal with shortcomings in your department, on your own terms, than to be subjected to an investigation instigated on the basis of a complaint by patients or staff. We have a professional duty to offer the best care and service delivery to our patients. Clinical audit is a useful tool to achieve this.

Finally, it will probably never be possible to convince everyone in the department of the value of undertaking a particular audit, so it is vital that anxieties are addressed from the start and everyone feels they can have their say. Clinical audit in physiotherapy may well encompass the tasks undertaken by support and administrative staff. It is vital they too are involved, from the outset, in any audit involving their work.

Brainstorming a topic for audit

Once staff are committed to the principles of clinical audit, topic brainstorming may begin. Topics for clinical audit may come from a variety of sources. They may be required by contractual agreement, arise from participation in a national or professional project, or be identified by problems in everyday practice. If you have a choice in what to audit, how do you decide what to start with?

Some physiotherapists spend a lot of time deciding on topics for audit, pulling ideas out of the air, and then judging whether they fit into departmental requirements. Although good ideas can often come from lateral thinking, most senior staff will have some inkling of areas of their service provision that could benefit from audit review. It may be useful to flag up potential audit suggestions along the structure, process and outcome lines, and to leave staff to consider their work in the light of those examples. More considered suggestions can then be discussed at the next staff meeting. The following examples of audit topics could be considered:

Structure

Equipment	Available electrotherapy equipment
Staff	Skill-mix, deployment, emergency cover
Training	Budget, in-service *versus* external courses
Working environment	Split sites, hotel/support services.

Process

Referrals	Referral patterns, GP *versus* consultant
Waiting lists	Time from referral to appointment, DNAs*
Documentation	Standard of note-keeping
Discharge procedures	Time from discharge to sending GP/consultant letter.

Outcome

Discharge patterns	Patients better *versus* referred back to GP/consultant
Re-referrals	No. of patients re-referred with same diagnosis

| Modality specific | Outcome and use of specific treatment, e.g. ice |
| Condition specific | Outcome of treatment in specific condition, e.g. shoulder capsulitis. |

These categories are expanded upon in later chapters.

*DNA, did not attend

Achieving a consensus

Choose a topic that fits one or more of the following categories (Crombie *et al.*, 1993):

- High risk
- High volume
- High cost
- Wide variation in clinical practice
- Local clinical anxiety.

For example, you may decide to choose a process audit of GP referrals because this is high volume and there is a wide variation in the quality of information on the referrals. The audit might be further stimulated by local anxiety that physiotherapists are unable to manage their workloads efficiently due to discrepancies in the information and urgency status indicated by GPs. The GPs may also have expressed concern that patients whom they consider need urgent treatment are being placed on a waiting list.

Another example may be an outcome audit to compare the efficacy of physiotherapy treatment of low back pain (high volume and wide variation in clinical practice) in the outpatient department with defined gold standards of clinical effectiveness (Waddell *et al.*, 1996). This audit would identify how closely actual intervention follows the set guidelines, and how many patients recover following treatment. A comparison follow-up audit, looking at the same issue in the community, might identify shortfalls in practice and highlight training requirements, or demonstrate a need for stricter clinical criteria for community *versus* outpatient treatment.

Formulate potential topic ideas into audit projects by looking back at the purpose of audit and ask the following questions:

- Will the results of this audit improve our knowledge of this aspect of service delivery?
- Can we use the results of this audit to optimize the quality, efficiency and effectiveness of our intervention or service delivery?
- Do we have the ability and the commitment to make the necessary changes indicated by the possible results of the audit?

Where staff identify several topics, prioritize according to the Crombie *et al.* (1993) guidelines and departmental need. Organize all the agreed topics into a rolling audit plan (see Chapter 4) taking care not to implement more than one at a time.

Once a topic has been agreed upon, the audit can begin.

Audit protocols

Audit protocols are not always mentioned in audit literature. The authors recommend the use of structured protocols to keep audit tasks on track, on time, and to ensure completion.

Audit protocols are similar to both research protocols and business plans in that they identify the aims and objectives, and the means by which these will be addressed. The protocol is also a statement of intent

Table 7.1   Audit protocol: Audit of physiotherapy records in outpatients

Problem statement: Clerical staff are increasingly concerned that physiotherapists are not collecting the necessary details on patient records, making it difficult to contact patients and their GPs. There is some concern that the necessary documentation standards are not being met.

Aim: To conduct an audit of randomly selected physiotherapy patient records.

Objective: To improve patient information recording on physiotherapy records.

Method: A note-keeping audit will be set up that can be used on a regular basis. Outpatient physiotherapy and administration staff will discuss and agree the standards and criteria to be used. The project manager has responsibility for identifying existing legal documentation requirements and the trust standards for documentation. The finalized data collection sheet will be used to audit a random sample of 30 physiotherapy patient records. The results of each audit will be reported to the staff at the monthly staff meeting. Any shortfalls in practice will be discussed and changes made where appropriate. It is anticipated that this will become a regular audit conducted by reception staff on a monthly basis.

Personnel

Project manager: (named) senior clerical officer, physiotherapy outpatients.
Data to be collected by: (named) receptionist.
Report to: (named) superintendent physiotherapist, physiotherapy outpatients.
Audit assistance available from: (named) audit assistant, trust audit department.

Timescale

Project manager to identify documentation standards (date).
Meeting to discuss audit set up, standards, criteria and data collection sheet (date).
*Audit department training of receptionist who will be collecting the data (date).
(*This will not always be necessary, especially if the audit is simple or the person responsible for data collection has previous audit experience.)
Data collection starts (date).
Data collection ends (date).
Project manager analyses data (date).
Report results to staff meeting (date).
Meeting to discuss implementation of changes (date).
Changes to be introduced at staff meeting (date).
Date of re-audit to ascertain change and improvement (date).

as to the reasons or need for the audit. In addition, it sets out the implications of undertaking such an audit, including costing, staff resources and a realistic time-scale.

The protocol does not need to be very long but it does need to be comprehensive, and it should be seen and agreed by all involved participants. It can then be used to keep the project on track. Specifically, it must clearly identify both time-scale and personnel. The project has a greater chance both of completion and achievement of its aims if it is clearly set out and agreed.

Table 7.1 is an example of an audit protocol.

Pre-audit surveys

Many physiotherapy audits are not true audits at all but rather pre-audit surveys of existing services. These surveys are important because they identify the baseline at which to set standards, which can then be used in a subsequent audit project. However, because they do not compare actual practice with any standards, they should not be considered as audits in their own right.

An example might be a survey such as that illustrated in Table 7.2, which examines the process of walking aid issue. Physiotherapy staff want to find out exactly what the process and problems are before setting any standards and auditing.

Table 7.2 Pre-audit survey: Survey of the process of issuing walking aids from the physiotherapy department

---

Problem statement: Walking aids are issued by clinicians and assistants. The paperwork is currently inefficient and incomplete. There is no effective system for tracking or recalling aids no longer in use by patients. The budget for walking aids is not keeping pace with demand.

Aims and objectives

1. To identify how many and what types of walking aids are being issued from the department.
2. To identify who is issuing them.
3. To identify why the current logging system is not functioning well.
4. To investigate the walking aids recall system.

Survey
Conduct a retrospective survey of walking aids issue looking back over the last six months in order to:

- Identify number and type of walking aids purchased by the department
- Identify number and type of walking aids held in department store
- Survey the logging system to identify who has issued what aid
- Survey the records to ascertain how many aids have been returned
- Survey the records to ascertain how many aids should be recalled.

The information obtained from such a survey can be used to inform standards for a subsequent audit. Formulating standards is considered in detail in the next chapter.

References

Crombie I.K., Davies H.T.O., Abraham S.C.S., Florey C. du V. (1993). *The Audit Handbook: Improving Health Care Through Clinical Audit.* John Wiley and Sons, Chichester.

Hartigan G. (1995). Clinical audit in animal therapy. *ACPAT Journal,* April.

Mann T. (1996). Clinical audit and its pivotal role in promoting clinical effectiveness. In *Clinical Audit in Context: The Role of Clinical Audit Within the Future Strategy of the NHS.* NHSE/NCCA Conference, Nottingham, 15 May, Conference Proceedings.

Standing Committee on Postgraduate Medical Education (1989). *Medical Audit: The Educational Complications.* SCOPME, London.

Waddell G., Feder G., McIntosh A., Lewis M., Hutchinson A. (1996). *Low Back Pain Evidence Review.* Royal College of General Practitioners, London.

Willmott M., Foster J., Walshe K., Coles J. (1995). *Evaluating Audit: A Review of Audit Activity in the Nursing and Therapy Professions.* Findings of a National Survey. CASPE Research, London.

8
Making audit work

Setting standards, defining criteria

General audit standards have already been considered in Chapter 4. This chapter looks at ways in which to identify standards relevant or specific to clinical audit in physiotherapy.

To audit a service or intervention, it is necessary to have standards against which to audit actual performance. The *Collins English Dictionary* defines a standard as an 'accepted example against which others are judged: a measure to which others must conform'.

Physiotherapists need to audit their practice against set standards. In some cases these standards will already have been set, in others it is up to clinicians to agree and set their own. There are four main types of standards used as benchmarks in audit:

- National
- Professional
- Corporate
- Internal.

National standards are agreed by national organizations and laid down for healthcare providers from a central or national level. Such standards include *The Patient's Charter* (HMSO, 1991), a Government initiative to improve the efficiency of healthcare provision. Other nationally set standards include those recommended by the Royal College of General Practitioners (Waddell *et al.*, 1996) such as standards for the treatment of patients with back pain. Standards are sometimes set internationally, such as those targets identified by the World Health Organization as part of its 'Health For All' initiative (WHO, 1985).

Professional standards are those that have been agreed by the professional bodies. Throughout the late 1980s and early 1990s, the Quality Assurance Working Party of the Chartered Society of Physiotherapy promoted the development of national guidelines and standards within the profession. Since then, many of the clinical interest groups within the Society have developed and published standards documents. A standards pack (CSP, 1993), including the *Standards of Physiotherapy Practice*, is available from the Professional Affairs Department of the CSP. The clinical interest group standards within the pack are revised every couple of years to keep up-to-date with current thinking and research. Other professional bodies have also developed guidelines and standards (e.g. The Royal College of Physicians' *Stroke Audit Package*, 1994) which may need to be taken into account when deciding standards for physiotherapy audit.

Corporate standards are devised at health service trust level and may relate to local *Patient's Charter* initiatives, local need and trust specialism. For example, trusts were obliged to devise their own specific standards based on *The Patient's Charter* in 1991. Many trusts published waiting list times for elective surgery or set specific standards for outpatient clinics. Trust standards may be set for every aspect of the service including hotel services, clinical specialism and managerial policy.

Internal standards are specifically designed to be used in individual audits and, as such, are entirely negotiated within the audit group (Crombie *et al.*, 1993). These must adhere to national, professional and corporate standards.

Drawing up standards and criteria for use in audit

Figure 8.1 shows the key components which should be considered when identifying or drawing up standards for any audit. A literature review will identify any existing standards, as well as up-to-date research which can inform evidence-based practice.

A standard is a formal statement of how patients should be managed (Crombie *et al.*, 1993). It should not be a 'wish list' only, but should contain achievable targets. Standards break down into criteria which are measurable (see Chapter 5). In fact it is the criteria which are measured or checked during an audit to see if a standard is being attained.

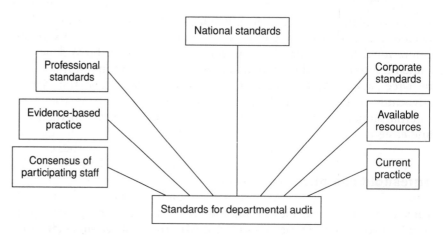

Figure 8.1 Key components which should be considered when setting standards

For example, a physiotherapy team may agree a standard that says, 'All referred patients will be assessed by a physiotherapist from the team within 3 days of receipt of the referral'. The criteria here are that:

- All referred patients will be assessed by a physiotherapist from the team.
- The assessment will be carried out within 3 days of receipt of referral.

These criteria can then be transferred to the audit data collection form as in Table 8.1

Table 8.1 Audit data collection form

Patient record	Assessed by physio YES/NO	Assessed within 3 days YES/NO
1.		
2.		
3. (etc.)		

Criteria which have a simple yes/no response are the easiest to use when analysing the audit data, as they are simple to code and calculate.

A useful method for deciding which criteria to use is the RUMBA method (Kitson *et al.*, 1990). The Royal College of Nursing (DySSSy) Standards of Care Project uses this to test the robustness of criteria (Malby, 1995). RUMBA is a mnemonic for:

Reliable – the criteria must be reliably and accurately identifiable and repeatable

Understandable – there must be no ambiguity as to how the criteria are interpreted

Measurable – it must be capable of being measured

Behavioural – it must relate to some behaviour or clinical significance (i.e. patient attended yes/no; patient better or worse)

Acceptable – it must be acceptable to all users of the criteria.

Standards and criteria are very much like 'the chicken and the egg'. You need to know what is going to be a measurable indicator of good quality before you define your standard, but you need to be able to break down the standard into measurable criteria in order to measure its application. The resource package *Moving to Audit* (Centre for Medical Education, 1995) advocates developing standards from criteria. When setting your own internal standards, there is no absolute rule. Use whichever method you find easiest.

Threshold compliance

Targets give you some idea of whether you can expect to achieve your standard 100% of the time. This is known as 'threshold compliance'. In a documentation audit, you may have standards that reflect legal obligations such as the requirement for the treating physiotherapist to sign the patient's records. This standard must achieve a 100% compliance, i.e. 100% of physiotherapy records audited will have the treating physiotherapist's signature. Other standards may be more difficult to achieve at a 100% threshold compliance. This may have nothing to do with the efficiency or effectiveness of the service or intervention; rather, it may reflect circumstances outside your control such as bank holidays interfering with arranging appointments, or unexpected complications in the pathology, or the social circumstances of the patient being treated.

Thresholds for compliance usually lie between 80% and 100% and reflect expectations based on previous experience and (sometimes) evidence-based practice. It is better to redefine standards more specifically than to accept a threshold for compliance of less than 80%.

For example, you may devise a standard for the treatment of people with back pain that states, 'All patients will be assessed within 1 week of receipt of referral – compliance threshold 60%'. This threshold is necessarily low because the standard does not distinguish between in-house and external referrals; neither does it distinguish between acute and chronic presentations, new patients or re-referrals. A 60% threshold tells you nothing. An audit that showed a 60% compliance lets you assume that everything is fine when there may be organizational improvements that could be made. It would be better to re-write the standard, possibly breaking it down into several standards, to obtain a better compliance threshold. Such new standards could read:

'All patients referred as new patients with acute low back pain will be assessed within 1 week of receipt of referral – 90%.'

'All new patients referred with non-urgent chronic low back pain will be assessed within 1 month of receipt of referral – 90%.'

These standards are far more realistic and will allow you to investigate the 10% shortfall on auditing to see if it is due to administrative overload, inefficiency or natural wastage (did not attend (DNA), unable to attend (UTA), change in degree of severity, etc.).

If you achieve your identified compliance threshold in your audit, consider upping the percentage, and thereby your expectations, to improve your service even more.

Exceptions

Some standards are written with exceptions. These are 'opt-out' clauses which further define the inclusion and exclusion criteria for the standard and may inform the level of threshold compliance.

For example, the following standard is described in an audit of inhaler use in an elderly care setting (used with permission):

Standard: 'All patients discharged home on respiratory inhalers will continue to demonstrate effective inhaler technique when checked 4–6 weeks post hospital discharge.'

Threshold compliance:	100%
Exceptions:	Re-admission to hospital
	Non-attendees to day hospital for review for audit purposes
	Death.

Identifying and choosing an appropriate audit tool

So many audits have already been undertaken that it seems ridiculous to 're-invent the wheel' by designing yet another audit data collection form. The central clinical audit department within your healthcare trust can be very helpful here. Many have standardized and computerized proformas for collecting the data needed in a notes audit, or a validated question-naire to obtain patient views of service delivery.

If you need to design a form from scratch, you will need to consider the following numbered points:

1. Will the audit gather data retrospectively or concurrently?
A concurrent audit will require clinicians or other staff members to col-lect data as they go along. This means producing a separate form for each data collector or for each patient. The forms will therefore need to be very 'user friendly' to facilitate compliance and easy completion. Annotation of the forms with notes on how to fill them in is very useful.

Table 8.2 shows an example of a concurrent audit data collection form for completion by the treating therapist. The treating physiotherapist may be asked to identify an appropriate set of records or to make some patient notes available, but the data collection is usually done by a physiotherapy assistant, clerical officer or clinical audit assistant. These forms are larger and more comprehensive and do not contain notes about how to fill them in, as the data collector will have received prior training.

Table 8.3 demonstrates an example of an audit form used in a retro-spective audit where a clinical audit assistant collects data from patient records. This illustrates an audit of postural advice to patients with low back pain. The audit assistant went through 300 randomly selected records of patients who had attended with back pain in the previous 9 months. Standards for postural correction and advice were in place prior to the audit. Note the differences in this form compared to Table 8.2. The audit assistant works though each patient record noting the relevant information on the data collection form.

2. Will the form give me the information I want?
This is an important question. It relates to both the quality and the quan-tity of the data collection sheet. There are two main rules here:

- Ask for the least possible amount of data that will still enable you to undertake your audit, i.e. compare actual practice with the set standards (content).
- Make sure you are asking the right questions (validity) in the right way (reliability).

Table 8.2   Audit data collection form for completion by treating therapist

---

Anytown Acute NHS Trust
Physiotherapy Department
Inpatient Elderly Care Audit

Thank you for taking part in this audit. We hope that the information gained will help to make our service more efficient by assessing the patients earlier in their stay.

Please attach one of these forms to each of your patient's records and complete it at the appropriate time. Completed forms to be handed to Fred in Physio Reception. Please start gathering data on Mon. 12th May. The audit ends on 14th June. Any questions to Sally, Supt. Physio, Day Hospital or bleep 123.

Patient's name ....
Date of birth ....
Date of admission ....
Date of physiotherapy assessment ....
Likely to benefit from physiotherapy treatment?: YES/NO *(please circle correct response)*
Physiotherapy treatment commenced (date) ....

Please note below any adverse incidents that may have prevented start of treatment such as falls or infection, etc.

Table 8.3   Posture audit data collection form

Patient index number	Site	Referral code	Posture correction recorded on exam. sheet	Posture correction recorded on POMR*	Patient using flexion or derangement noted	Lateral shift noted	McKenzie Institute form used	Other form used	No form used

*POMR, problem-oriented medical record.

Content

Do not be tempted to ask 'just one more question as that looks interesting'. Too many boxes to tick or questions to answer will irritate some and cause others to fabricate. In a traffic survey undertaken by children outside their school, one hour in particular appeared to have such heavy traffic that the teacher questioned why there was not gridlock. Further investigation showed that bored school boys on the afternoon shift got fed up with counting vehicles and ticked boxes according to how many wheels went by, not how many cars! It is not unknown for similar fabrications to occur in both audit and research.

Even if all your returned data are accurate, what are you going to do with the results? Collect enough data to complete the task in hand only.

Validity

Ensure that the questions you ask and the data you collect are valid. Are you asking the right question? Will the answer give you the information you require? Are you recording what you intended? Validity is a complex subject, which involves both the construction of the form and choice of any measurement tools (Bowling, 1991), and is considered further, in the context of outcome measurement, in Chapter 11. Covering all elements of the subject is beyond the scope of this book, and further information may be gleaned from research methods or health measurement books.

Reliability

Drawing up a data collection sheet is often fine until you come to fill it in. Unless the form can be consistently and identically filled in both over time and by different people, then the information it collects will be un-reliable. The form therefore needs to be accurate and precise enough to ensure that two people filling in the same form for the same situation (e.g. patient record or administrative procedure) would complete it in an identical fashion. The form also needs to be robust over time. That is, it contains enough instruction to enable a single assessor to complete two forms about the same situation accurately, despite having a time lapse between completion. More information about reliability is given in Chapter 11, and also in research methods and health measurement texts (e.g. Bowling, 1991).

3. Should I test the audit form before I use it?
Any data collection form should be piloted prior to application. This will check for several things:

- Acceptability within the department
- Validity of the content
- Ambiguous questions
- Inaccurate or incomplete instructions
- Ease of use
- As an indicator of the time it will take to complete
- Pilot data can be analysed to see if you are asking the right questions.

Pilot data should not be entered into the main audit. Unlike some research, in clinical audit the data collection sheets can be piloted on the clinicians who will be completing the real thing and on part of the main cohort, e.g. patient records, administrative procedure.

4. Should I select a random sample of records, procedures or patients for my audit?

Clinical audit differs from research in that it seeks to evaluate actual practice – warts and all. Most research projects select their subject cohort very carefully, taking all sorts of inclusions and exclusions into consideration. It is true that your cohort must reflect your standard. For example, it would be unrealistic to conduct a total hip replacement audit in the paediatric department! However, sheer numbers may require you to audit only a sample of your practice rather than the whole.

Note-keeping audits are a good example of this. If you wish to undertake an audit of the completeness of patient records, you will need to set some parameters. For example you may choose to define a time scale, a single unit from within the department and a set number of records:

Time scale:	Records from patients discharged in June
Unit:	Cardiothoracic surgery physiotherapy team
Records:	10 randomly selected records from each physiotherapist on the team.

5. Do I need ethical approval?

In general terms, clinical audit does not require ethical approval (see Chapter 5). Clinical audit simply evaluates current practice and does not seek to manipulate either subject or methodology. However, audit in some very sensitive areas (such as sending patient satisfaction questionnaires to seriously ill patients) or of vulnerable patient groups, such as those with profound learning disabilities or those with mental health problems, may require ethical approval. If you are in any doubt, obtain advice from the trust clinical audit department or local research ethics committee. These committees are based in health authorities and cover their geographic area regardless of whether the research is being conducted within the NHS, private, independent or charitable sector, or through an academic establishment.

Completing the audit

We have already noted that many audits do not reach completion and that this is a waste of time and resources, as well a source of disillusionment for participating staff. Three ways to ensure that an audit project is satisfactorily completed are to allocate a named audit project leader, to set a time scale and to write and distribute an agreed protocol (see Chapter 7). Another aide memoire is to attach an audit cycle tick box list to all paperwork dealing with a particular audit, as illustrated in Table 8.4. This allows participants and managers to see at a glance where you are up to in the audit cycle, and acts as a reminder to revisit the audit once changes in

Table 8.4   Audit progress sheet

Title of audit:	
Observe practice	☐
Set standards	☐
Collect data (audit)	☐
Compare practice with standards (analyse audit data)	☐
Identify necessary improvements	☐
Suggest changes	☐
Implement changes	☐
Evaluate changes (re-audit)	☐
Review standards	☐

(Used with permission.)

practice have been made. The boxes can be ticked and dated as the audit progresses.

References

Bowling A. (1991). *Measuring Health: A Review of Quality of Life Measurement Scales*. Open University Press, Milton Keynes.

Centre for Medical Education, University of Dundee and CRAG, Scotland. (1995). *Moving to Audit*. University of Dundee, Scotland.

Chartered Society of Physiotherapy (1993). *Standards of Physiotherapy Practice*, 2nd edn. 14 Bedford Row, London W1R 4ED.

Crombie I.K., Davies H.T.O., Abraham S.C.S., Florey C. du V. (1993). *The Audit Handbook: Improving Health Care Through Clinical Audit*. John Wiley and Sons, Chichester.

HMSO (1991). *The Patient's Charter*. HMSO, London.

Kitson A., Hyndman W., Harvey G., Yerrell P. (1990). *Quality Patient Care: The Dynamic Standard Setting System*. Scutari Press, London.

Malby B. (ed.) (1995). *Clinical Audit for Nurses and Therapists*. Scutari Press, London.

Royal College of Physicians of London (1994). *Stroke Audit Package*. 11 St. Andrew's Place, London NW1 4LE

Waddell G., Feder G., McIntosh A., Lewis M., Hutchinson A. (1996). *Low Back Pain Evidence Review*. Royal College of General Practitioners, London.

World Health Organization (1985). *Targets for Health for All*. WHO, Copenhagen.

9

Structure audit in physiotherapy

Chapter 3 has already considered the theory of choosing a topic for clinical audit of structure. This chapter looks at the practicalities of designing, applying and interpreting structure audits in physiotherapy. Examples of structure audits are considered.

To recap, structure, according to Donabedian (1966), comprises the actual structure or 'hardware' of an organization. It comprises all the structural elements that make up the framework of the establishment and includes the buildings and facilities, the equipment, staff numbers, skills and skill-mix. Other things that relate to the smooth operation of the organization, such as its support systems for administration, pay and training, all come under the heading of structure.

The physiotherapy department may be subject to structure audits that are not run by physiotherapists themselves. For example, the domestic department may run continuous or concurrent audits of cleanliness in the patient waiting areas and cloakrooms that service the physiotherapy department. They will have predetermined standards of hygiene that are checked in random audits.

Example 1

Physiotherapists managing an outpatient department can conduct spot audits to see if physiotherapy equipment is up to standard, as in example 1 (Table 9.1). The audit data collection form illustrated in Table 9.2 is used.

The superintendent in the outpatient department asked the physiotherapy assistant to gather this information and the results are set out in Table 9.3.

This type of audit is all about ensuring that the necessary resources are in place to facilitate service delivery. It is not about catching people out when they borrow equipment in an emergency. However, unless everyone in the department appreciates this, such an exercise can look as if blame is being apportioned. It is the responsibility of the manager to ensure that everyone is involved and understands the reason for the audit from the outset.

Table 9.1 Structure audit of equipment availability and safety

Venue: Physiotherapy outpatient department

Standards

1. The following items of electrical equipment are situated in the department at all times:

   - Ultrasound machine × 3
   - Interferential × 2
   - Pulsed short-wave × 1
   - Laser unit × 1
   - Electrical stimulation unit × 1
   - TNS* for demonstration (not for loan) × 1.

2. All electrical equipment will have a sticker noting the date of the last and next due maintenance service; to include the above list plus the ice machine.
3. None of the electrical equipment noted above will have an out-of-date maintenance sticker.

Criteria

Standard 1: Equipment – present/absent
Standard 2: Service sticker correctly completed – yes/no
Standard 3: Date of next service later than today's date – yes/no

Threshold for compliance: 100%

TNS, transcutaneous nerve stimulation.

Table 9.2 Audit data collection form

Date of audit:			
Electrical equipment	Criteria		
	Present/absent	Service sticker?	Date of next service
Ultrasound 1			
Ultrasound 2			
Ultrasound 3			
Interferential 1			
Interferential 2			
Pulsed short-wave			
Laser			
Electrical stimulator			
TNS*			
Ice machine			

*TNS, transcutaneous nerve stimulation.

Table 9.3   Results of spot audit

Standard 1: One ultrasound machine was missing, the TNS machine was missing.

Standard 2: All equipment present had an appropriate service label attached.

Standard 3: All equipment present except the electrical stimulator achieved this standard.

Action

1. Identify why some equipment was missing. *The ultrasound was found on the orthopaedic wards as their machine was faulty. The TNS had been given to a patient as the loan machines were all out.*
2. Identify why the electrical stimulator had not been serviced. *It was found that the suppliers had ceased trading and no contingency plans had been made for servicing.*
3. Rectify these points and re-audit without warning within the next 3 months.

Changes

1. Staff to be informed about systems for reporting and replacing faulty equipment at next staff meeting.
2. Senior staff to survey case notes to identify from clinical need how many TNS machines should be available for loan. Staff to be reminded that the departmental TNS is not to be loaned.
3. Manager to investigate equipment servicing contracts and ensure that all equipment is covered.

It is also important that managers are seen to act on the results to improve the efficiency of the department. Nothing causes more disinclination towards undertaking subsequent projects than failure to act on the results of the previous audit.

The advantage of this type of audit is that, once the standards have been agreed, the audit can be undertaken quickly and helps to improve the efficiency of the department. It can also be quickly and easily repeated at regular intervals. In addition, it has the advantage of raising awareness amongst staff about the importance of ensuring all equipment is regularly serviced, and identifies the correct procedures for reporting faulty or missing equipment.

Example 2

Other areas of structure that can be audited include skill-mix. A busy community physiotherapy service was finding its staff resources spread thinner as the workload increased. There was some concern that physiotherapy assistants were undertaking tasks that should have been done by qualified staff. Similarly, qualified staff felt that much of their time was being taken up with clerical tasks. The audit is summarized in Table 9.4.

Strictly speaking, this project was a pre-audit survey and not a true audit as the actual practice noted was not compared with any standards. How-

Table 9.4   Structure audit of skill-mix in the community

Background:	Need to identify working practices and optimize staff deployment.
Venue:	A domiciliary physiotherapy service in a mainly rural, elderly setting.
Method:	All physiotherapy and physiotherapy assistant staff were asked to keep a record of the clinical and administrative tasks they undertook during one working week, together with working and travelling time. For each identified task, staff were asked to say whether they felt this was most appropriate to be undertaken by a qualified physiotherapist or a physiotherapy assistant.
Results:	22 different treatment and administrative tasks were identified. At a meeting of all domiciliary physiotherapy staff, each task was considered separately as to whether it required the skill and expertise of a qualified therapist or whether it should safely and effectively be undertaken by a trained physiotherapy assistant. 16 tasks were identified.

Review of results
Following this audit, physiotherapy assistants were trained and employed within the domiciliary service to carry out the appropriate identified tasks. A re-audit confirmed a saving of qualified physiotherapy time equal to 16% of the total hours worked in the community.

(Used with permission.)

ever, local standards emerged from this survey and were used to re-audit the service several months later. National professional guidelines such as those published by the CSP (1994) relating to the management of physiotherapy assistants are useful benchmarks for setting standards.

Other examples of physiotherapy structure audit

- Training courses, their availability and uptake by staff
- Emergency on-call procedures
- Staff use of continuing professional development diary
- Staffing levels on the wards during school holiday periods
- Acupuncture equipment health and safety procedures
- Individual performance review (IPR) system.

References

Chartered Society of Physiotherapy (1994). *Guidelines for the Management of Physiotherapy Helpers*. 14 Bedford Row, London WC1R 4ED.
Donabedian A. (1966). *Evaluating the Quality of Medical Care*. Millbank Memorial Federation of Quality, USA. Part 3, pp. 166–203.

10
Process audit in physiotherapy

Physiotherapy process audit is concerned with all aspects of the process of physiotherapy service. It includes all those processes whereby patients get into, through and out of the system. Sitting between structure and outcome, process audits frequently shift across the boundaries. In particular, the 'hands on' aspect of physiotherapy intervention and treatment is pertinent to both audit of process and audit of outcome. For example, auditing the appropriateness of methods of treatment offered for a specific condition, based on agreed standards or published research on treatment for that condition, would be regarded as an audit of process. This is different from an audit which identifies whether the health outcome of physiotherapy treatment for a specific condition achieves set standards (audit of outcome). The difference is in the way in which the standards are set. In the first example, the standards refer to whether the methods of treatment in practice follow published recommendations on methods of treatment appropriate to that condition. In the latter example, the standards refer to whether the health outcome achieved for patients with a specific condition matches the expected outcome after physiotherapy intervention for that condition, as based on research literature.

It was stated in Chapter 3 that the most effective audits are likely to consider elements of structure, process and outcome as part of the same project. Thus, structure, process and outcome should be seen as loose categorizations of health service audit and as a means to ensure that clinicians audit all aspects of service delivery systematically, rather than concentrating on 'pockets' of quality in some areas to the detriment of others. However, for the purposes of simplicity, this book offers discrete examples of structure, process and outcome audit, which can be built upon and combined as experience of clinical audit increases in individual physiotherapists and departments.

Process audits are probably the most common audits undertaken in physiotherapy departments. This is because they are relatively easy and gather a lot of information which can inform service delivery. Naturally, it takes time and application to set up a process audit for the first time but, once a satisfactory audit has been tried and tested, it can be used regularly and repeatedly for as long as that process remains in force.

Setting up a process audit

1. Deciding what to audit

Looking back at Chapter 7, and the criteria used for deciding what to audit, it is necessary to decide if any particular area of service delivery falls into one of the categories described. Processes set up within the department to facilitate service delivery are unlikely to be of high risk, but some may well be of high volume or high cost. You cannot audit everything at once, so choose something that you consider to be achievable, and something where you know you will be able to make service improvements based on the results of the audit. You may also be under pressure from health service trust managers or purchasers to audit one particular area of service delivery as part of a wider service evaluation.

Consider the processes that make up your physiotherapy service. These include the processes by which patients hear about your service, and get into, through and out of the system. Identify the parts that go to make up each particular process. For example, when looking at the process of how patients get into the system you will need to ask yourself the following:

- Are patients referred by hospital consultants, GPs, other health professionals, self-referred?
- What systems are in place to process these referrals?
- Do you have the same system for all, or does it vary either according to the referral source or between different units within your department?
- Are all staff aware of the systems?
- Are they following the correct procedures?
- Are your systems as efficient as they could be?

After departmental discussion, senior staff usually have the final say over what is audited.

2. Getting a process audit started

Having identified which area of service delivery is to be audited, the next task is to set up the project.

- Designate an audit project manager who will be responsible for setting up and running the audit.
- Identify any standards that need to be used in this audit. These may be pre-existing standards from a previous audit, national guidelines or trust standards. A literature review will identify further research evidence upon which to base standards.
- Decide whether the audit data can be collected retrospectively or if a concurrent audit needs to be performed.
- Invite everyone who has any input into the service that is being audited into discussions about finalizing the standards and criteria to be used, deciding the format of the audit data collection and choosing the most appropriate time to undertake the audit.
- Pilot the audit form to see if it is feasible to collect the data you seek – poor information recording in medical records may make a retrospective

audit almost impossible in some cases. Check that the data collection form is not ambiguous and can be reliably completed by different people on different days if necessary. Also ensure that you are collecting the right information that will tell you whether or not standards are being met.

3. Running a process audit

When everyone involved is happy with the audit method and time-frame, standards and data collection sheet, you can start the actual project.

- Ensure everyone involved knows that the audit is happening, when it starts and ends, and what their responsibilities are regarding completing audit data collection sheets.
- Clinical audit should not significantly interfere with the process it seeks to evaluate. An audit should help to streamline a process in the long run without hindering it in the short term.
- The project manager should keep a close eye on the running of the audit and be available to cope with unexpected hiccoughs.

4. Using the audit data

Once the audit data gathering is complete, the information can be analysed to see if actual practice meets set standards.

- Analyse the audit information
- Identify where standards are being met
- Identify where standards are not being met
- Write a short report for staff who are affected by the results of the audit
- You may also need to write a report for trust managers or purchasers if you have undertaken the audit for them.

5. Completing the cycle

Running the audit project and feeding back to staff is not enough if the audit cycle is to be completed.

- Discuss the findings of the audit with all involved staff
- Where standards have been met, ask if standards could be raised to increase efficiency further
- Where standards have not been met, discuss how the process could be refined to optimize the quality and efficiency of this particular process
- Obtain a commitment to make the changes necessary to reach the set standards
- Plan to re-audit in the future
- Re-audit.

The theory of audit identifies a logical process. The practice of audit can be fraught with practical problems. The examples which follow are all real physiotherapy process audits (used with permission). They all follow the audit process and their results identify areas where the quality and efficiency of service provision could be improved. In addition, practical problems encountered with the actual audit process are identified. The reader is invited to consider the reality of conducting audits, and to compare it with his or her own experiences where appropriate.

Example I

Title
Audit of GP discharge letters.

Background
The physiotherapy department business plan required senior staff to undertake audits of patient records to see if they adhered to quality assurance initiatives.

Method
Copies of all GP discharge summaries completed over a month in a physiotherapy outpatient department were collected. These were reviewed independently, against set criteria, by a superintendent physiotherapist from a sister department and another independent physiotherapy assistant. Each letter was scrutinized to determine whether the criteria were present, absent or not applicable. Standards were set at 100% compliance for each criterion. The project was managed by the superintendent physiotherapist in the outpatient department.

Results
62 letters were examined against the criteria below and the data are set out in Table 10.1.

Review of audit data collection form
Although the form had been piloted, further room for improvement was noted:

- Point number 9 could be subdivided into subjective and objective.
- Definition of the term legible (point 14) – this could be subdivided into 'readable' and 'understandable'.

Review of audit process
The project manager (the superintendent physiotherapist) identified several problems with the setting up and running of the actual audit. These included:

- Getting staff members to agree and define the criteria to be used in the audit.
- The audit was perceived to have a low degree of importance due to other constraints present within the department, including annual leave, workload and waiting times.

Table 10.1   Audit results of GP discharge letters

Letter content – criteria	Data present	Data absent	Not applicable
1. Patient's name	61 (98%)	1 (2%)	0
2. Date of birth	60 (97%)	2 (3%)	0
3. Patient's address	61 (98%)	1 (2%)	0
4. Hospital where treated	54 (87%)	8 (13%)	0
5. Therapist's name	22 (36%)	40 (64%)	0
6. Date referral letter received in dept.	6 (10%)	56 (90%)	0
7. Date of first treatment	37 (60%)	25 (40%)	0
8. Number of treatment contacts	41 (66%)	21 (34%)	0
9. Findings on examination	37 (60%)	25 (40%)	0
10. Treatment modality	47 (76%)	15 (24%)	0
11. Outcome recorded			
(a) Subjective	13 (21%)	49 (79%)	0
(b) Objective	46 (74%)	14 (23%)	2 (3%)
12. Future action/plan	61 (98%)	1 (2%)	0
13. Signature	62 (100%)	0	0
14. Letter legible	39 (63%)	20 (32%)	3 (5%)

- Time spent by the superintendents and assistant on the project.

Review of audit results

Despite the problems identified within the audit process, the actual audit results were felt to give useful information. The following were the key problems highlighted by the audit:

- Different discharge letter formats had resulted in inconsistent content of discharge summaries.
- Recording the date of receipt of referral letter was not found to be relevant.
- Vital information (patient's name, address, date of birth) was missing in 7%.
- Although all discharge summaries were signed, only 36% also had the therapist's name written legibly.
- Objective signs were often ambiguous, for example range of movement (ROM) was not defined as to whether it indicated active or passive, and on some occasions the joint being referred to was not identified.
- Use of abbreviations and jargon was common, e.g. u/s, mob., NAGS and SNAGS.

Actions and recommendations

The results of the audit were presented at a staff meeting. Following discussion, various decisions were made, including:

- Implementation of guidelines for a model discharge summary letter
- Re-audit in 3 months' time without prior warning
- Amending the audit form in the light of the audit form review

- Ensuring patient details (sticky label) are attached to each summary
- Heightening awareness and commitment to audit amongst staff in keeping with the physiotherapy business plan
- Heightening purchasers' awareness of the time, cost and staff resources needed to initiate, conduct and disseminate the findings of audit.

Example 2

This example again looks at documentation, this time to see if it adhered to national standards set by a physiotherapy specific interest group.

Title
An audit of physiotherapy records of patients with respiratory conditions.

Background
Documentation standards were set by the Association of Chartered Physiotherapists in Respiratory Care. This audit sought to identify whether these standards were being adhered to in practice by the physiotherapy respiratory team in a district general hospital.

Method
The standards were identified from the CSP standards file. Each physio-therapist on the team supplied his or her last ten patient records for audit. The following documentation requirements were established from the standards and used as criteria in the audit:

- History of present condition
- Smoking
- Breathing pattern
- Palpation
- Auscultation
- X-ray findings
- Full signature of therapist
- A measurable goal.

Results
These showed 40% compliance with the standards. Particular gaps were:

- Breathing pattern
- Palpation
- X-ray findings.

Review of audit results

- Team meeting to discuss the findings
- Further in-service training on standards
- Need for an assessment sheet specifically designed for ventilated patients.

Further documentation was re-audited a few months later.

Re-audit results

- Forty seven per cent compliance to standards. Documentation of palpation and X-ray findings remained a weakness.
- Although the assessment sheet was well used, the team was to meet to discuss changes to improve compliance with documentation standards.

Example 3

Not all process audits are documentation audits. Process includes the ways that patients enter, move through and leave the system. The following example looks at an audit of waiting times within a physiotherapy outpatient department (used with permission).

Background

This audit was chosen as the department has a large through-put of patients. It was not known whether the waiting times either for an appointment, or in the clinic itself, were up to standard.

Audit aim

To determine whether the department was meeting present standards for 'waiting times'.

Standards

Standards were already set based on national guidelines, trust standards and the physiotherapy department business plan. Clinical and clerical staff were aware of the standards. The following standards were in use for routine and non-urgent cases. Other standards were in place for urgent referrals but these were not being audited. The pre-set standards were as follows:

- That 100% of patients will receive an appointment date which is less than or equal to 10 working days from the date that referral was received in the physiotherapy department.
- That 90% of patients will be seen within 15 minutes of the time stated on the appointment card.

To ensure clarity, waiting times were further defined as follows:

- The number of working days between the date the referral arrived in the physiotherapy department and the date of appointment for physiotherapy. This did not include the actual day the referral arrived, and the next working day counted as day 1.
- The time spent by a patient waiting to be called in for treatment after the time stated on the appointment card. Waiting time spent by patients who arrived early was not included.

Table 10.2   Patient questionnaire

1. Have you been treated by a physiotherapist at this hospital before?

    Yes ☐   No ☐

2. Do you consider your condition to be urgent?

    Yes ☐   No ☐

3. How many working days did you expect to wait until the date of your first appointment (from the day your referral arrived in the physiotherapy department)?

    .... *days*

4. How many minutes did you expect to wait between your appointment time and actually seeing the physiotherapist?

    .... *minutes*

5. How many minutes did you actually wait after your appointment time before

    .... *minutes*

Method

A start date was agreed and the next 100 consecutive referrals were used in the audit. Reception staff recorded the date the referrals arrived in the department and the number of working days between that date and the appointment date. Each of the 100 patients received a letter with the appointment card asking them to complete a questionnaire (Table 10.2) and hand it to the treating physiotherapist.

Results

- A response rate of 46 (46%) was achieved.
- Answers to the five questions were analysed:

    Question 1.   Percentage having previous physiotherapy: 41.3%
    Question 2.   Percentage considering themselves 'urgent': 56.5%
    Question 3.   Mean expected number of working days before the appointment date: 18.4 days
    Question 4.   Mean expected number of minutes between appointment time and treatment: 17.5 minutes
    Question 5.   Mean actual number of minutes between the appointment time and treatment: 4.0 minutes

    Mean actual number of working days before the appointment date (noted by the reception staff): 10.1 days.

- Patients who considered themselves 'urgent' expected to wait, on average, 16.6 days. They actually waited 9.5 days. These patients expected, on average, to wait 17.8 minutes past their appointed time but actually only waited 2.9 minutes.

- Patients who considered themselves to be 'non-urgent' expected to wait, on average, 20.7 days and actually waited 11 days. Similarly, these patients expected to wait, on average, 17.1 minutes and actually waited an average of 5.4 minutes past their appointed time.
- Expected waiting times were very similar between new and previously attending patients.
- Revisiting the standards, it can be seen that 47.8% of patients were not seen within 10 working days and therefore failed to meet the required standard.
- However, no patient had to wait 15 or more minutes for treatment after their appointed time, achieving a 100% adherence to this standard.

Review of audit results

- The physiotherapists and reception staff felt that this audit had been a useful exercise undertaken at minimum effort and cost.
- It was felt important to have gathered information on whether patients were new or previous attendees as this may have had some bearing on expectations based on prior knowledge, although this appears not to have been the case.
- 56.5% of patients considered their condition in urgent need of treatment. It was decided to compare this perception to the treating physiotherapist's assessment in a future audit.
- Actual waiting times in the department were less than patients' expectations. This was felt to promote a positive image of the department.
- An investigation into the failure to achieve the first standard showed that there was an unusually high level of staff annual leave over this period and a change in junior post rotation. Staff agreed to investigate this problem further and develop some recommendations for discussion at a future staff meeting.
- Standard 1 was discussed by the staff group. A proposal was put forward to amend it, in the light of current staffing levels, as this level of service could not presently be guaranteed to purchasers or patients. (NB This demonstrates an example of audit of process shifting towards audit of structure, as staffing levels are regarded as part of the structure of an organization.)

Re-audit

The superintendent physiotherapist undertaking this audit advised staff that a re-audit would take place 6 months after new standards were implemented, and following agreement from trust managers and purchasers.

Other examples of physiotherapy process audits

- Referral patterns
- Clinician/reception staff communication procedures
- Waiting times for specialist referral, e.g. hydrotherapy or back school
- Waiting lists at peak times and holiday periods

- Response times for emergency physiotherapy
- Specialist/generalist clinician workload
- Appropriateness of intervention for a specific condition.

11
Outcome measurement

The preceding two chapters dealt with the practicalities of setting up structure and process audits of physiotherapy practice. The next chapter deals in the same way with physiotherapy audit of outcome. Outcome audit differs slightly from structure and process audit in that it is the aspect of clinical audit which relies most heavily upon research evidence, and for which there is a greater need to develop standards based on the clinical literature and up-to-date research findings. Reliable outcome measurement is crucial in this category of audit, and it is advisable for clinicians to familiarize themselves with the concept of outcome measurement, and to consider some of the many measures available, before embarking upon an audit of outcome. The current chapter is therefore devoted to outcome measurement, both in general and specific to physiotherapy clinical audit.

The outcome of treatment for an episode of care may be measured using outcome measures.

Outcome measures are currently used in three main areas:

1. In contracting, where commissioners may use evidence of good outcome of treatment as an indicator of where to purchase. (Long, 1994)
2. By clinicians, in day-to-day assessment of patients to ascertain the extent of their problems and the effect that changing pathology and/or intervention is having. This can be used as a measure of clinical effectiveness.
3. In research, where robust, valid and reliable outcome indicators are vital to ascertain the value of a particular intervention.

Clinical audit of outcome is usually undertaken to assure clinicians, their managers and/or commissioners that their interventions are timely, appropriate and effective. Increasingly, outcome audits are being undertaken to test adherence to clinical guidelines.

Outcome definitions

Outcomes are defined as:

- 'The results (effects) of processes. They are that part of the situation pertaining after a process which can be attributed to the process.' (*Outcomes Briefing*, 1993)

- 'Health outcomes are the effects on health of any type of process.' (*Outcomes Briefing*, 1993)

Health outcomes can also be defined as:

- 'A change in the health of an individual, a group of people or a population which is attributable to an intervention or a series of interventions.' (New South Wales Department of Health, 1992)

A physiotherapy outcome measure can be defined as:

- 'A measurement against which the alteration in health status of a patient, that is likely to be due to physiotherapy intervention, can be judged.' (Barnard, 1993)

Three main points are common to each of these definitions:

1. There is a result or outcome from the process
2. That outcome is measurable
3. The outcome is attributable to that process or intervention.

Obtaining a result

When we treat patients, we do so for a reason. Classically, the patient attends with a physical health problem for which he or she is seeking relief and, hopefully, resolution. The patient and the therapist keep a close eye on the progress of the treatment, looking for signs of improvement.

An outcome measure is more than just a result. When you take an exam you are informed of the result. The result may be simply pass or fail or it may be graded or given a numeric score. Results can be listed in a hierarchical way; for example in the Government's league tables for schools. Such lists can be used to see how results change from year to year and may have a wider influence on how students are trained. However, to the student, passing the exam means much more than the result. The outcome of the training course may partly be the exam result, but it is also the skills acquired and knowledge gained. Therefore the outcome is the result plus the experience that took place during the process that led to the result. When you pass your driving test, you not only receive a full driving licence (the result), you also have the competency and skills to drive (the outcome).

A patient receiving physiotherapy for an acute back problem may see returning to work as a satisfactory result of treatment. However the outcome encompasses the effect of the whole process of intervention, including relief of pain, return to function, and advice and education to reduce recurrence.

Obtaining outcomes that are measurable

By definition, an outcome measure must be measurable. Outcomes can have: a quantifiable component, e.g. range of movement; a qualitative component, e.g. subjective impression of pain; or a combination of both, e.g. walking can be measured in terms of quantity (distance) and quality (normal gait pattern). Measuring outcomes in physiotherapy is considered more fully later in this chapter.

Attribution

Many processes influence health. Disease is an obvious one, but health is also influenced by a number of other factors including housing, the environment, social class and wealth (Whitehead, 1988). The key to measuring outcome is the issue of attribution. This is always a problem when measuring any health outcome, as both health and disease are continuously fluctuating states. If a patient arrives in an outpatient department with a sprained ankle, how can you show that your intervention is the reason for his recovery and return to the football pitch within a few weeks? An elderly man may be admitted to the ward with an exacerbation of his chronic obstructive pulmonary disease and returns home much improved a couple of weeks later. Is this due to a spontaneous recovery now he is out of his damp flat and not allowed to smoke? Are the good nursing and revamped drug regimes key factors? How much effect, if any, did your hours of physiotherapy treatment have on the final outcome?

A young woman with multiple sclerosis is visited by the community physiotherapist. She feels much better for her treatment and her husband has learnt how to transfer her safely. However, the disease process means that, physically, she is worse at the end of the course of treatment than she was at the start. Everyone agrees that your intervention has had a good outcome, but how can this be shown?

There is no easy answer to the issue of attribution. Only rigorous randomized controlled research trials, conducted at multiple centres with large numbers of subjects, can ever show true outcomes of intervention. Physiotherapists use the findings of such research to treat a patient in the belief that the treatment will have the desired outcome. Clinical audit checks whether this belief is well founded. Do not forget that clinical audit looks at *actual* practice in a *specific* setting, in order to match what is happening in reality to the standards you wish to achieve. It is important, however, to be aware of attribution and not to make sweeping claims about physiotherapy outcomes in audit.

Choosing outcome measures

The Chartered Society of Physiotherapy recommends that, where possible, physiotherapists use pre-existing validated health measurement scales as outcome measures, as these have been shown to have degrees of validity and reliability (CSP, 1995).

When choosing an outcome measure, remember that it should be valid, reliable, appropriate and responsive enough to use in a particular situation. The concept of validity refers to the extent to which a test measures what it is intended to measure (McDowell and Newell, 1996) and the extent to which one's findings are accurate and reflect the purpose of the investigation (DePoy and Gitlin, 1993). Validity is described by le Roux in terms of the potential for bias in the measuring scale used to measure outcome. He states: 'The effect of bias is a measure of the validity of an outcome of a measuring procedure, and shows the extent to which the description provided by the measuring process is correct, and therefore a true description of the attribute under consideration.' (le Roux, 1997)

In other words, choose the right outcome for the right condition. Return to work may be an entirely appropriate outcome measure to use for a young, self-employed man receiving physiotherapy for an acute back condition. It would not be an appropriate outcome measure to use for an unemployed man with chronic back pain attending back school classes. Also ensure that measurement of the outcome is accurate. Beware of using valid outcome measuring procedures in inappropriate situations, as this will invalidate the entire outcome measure, e.g. using ability to climb stairs as an indicator of function in patients with chronic obstructive pulmonary disease where this may more accurately reflect their cardiac condition rather than any improvement in their lung function.

Many existing health measurement scales, such as the Barthel score, have been developed and standardized for certain groups of people. This index has been shown to be 'capable of successfully predicting mortality, length of hospital stay and progress amongst stroke patients' (Bowling, 1991). It is therefore felt to report some predictive validity. Note, however, that this predictive validity applies only to the use of the index for adults with stroke. Its validity in other groups is not necessarily proven.

Validity is a complex subject, having many different components which fall outside the scope of this book. Readers are referred to texts dealing with health measurement scales which identify the validity and reliability of individual health measurement scales (Bowling, 1991 and 1995; Cole et al., 1995; McDowell and Newell, 1996; Wade, 1992). It should be noted that some health measurement scales have been standardized using relatively small numbers of subjects, which may limit their validity.

'Reliability' is defined as consistency and dependability (McDowell and Newell, 1996). Outcome measures must have this quality in order to be robust. The parameters of the measure must be laid down so that they are accurately repeatable, not just by one therapist but by any who may conduct the measurement. When using fluctuation in swelling as an outcome measure, it is important to specify how and where this is measured and so ensure repeatability by any therapist. Unfortunately, many outcome measures lack reliability due to inherent ambiguities in the format of the questions. A question in the Rivermead mobility index regarding turning over in bed asks, 'Do you turn over from your back to your side without help?' The scoring is a simple Yes/No. Yet two physiotherapists asking the same patient scored different answers. The patient replied, 'I can sometimes, but I need someone to replace the bed covers after I have turned.' One therapist interpreted this as 'Yes', as the patient could, on occasion, perform the task of turning on the bed. The other therapist said

'No' because the patient could not perform the task every time and needed some secondary help. Without clearer instructions, this simple question becomes ambiguous and affects the reliability of the test. Almost all outcome measures, both pre-existing and home-grown, have the potential to be unreliable. Always examine them very carefully to ensure that they are reliable and can be interpreted consistently by all who will be using them.

'Appropriate' is defined as suitable or fitting. It may be entirely appropriate to use high-tech lung function equipment in a hospital setting to measure the outcome of treatment for chronic respiratory disease, but totally inappropriate in the community setting where the necessary equipment is not readily available. If you are choosing outcome measures for audit of a complete episode of care, it is important to choose measures that can be used in all the necessary settings.

'Responsive' is defined as sensitive, reacting readily. A responsive outcome measure will indicate the changes you require. The Barthel Index is widely used to monitor functional independence. It has been found to be a useful scale for monitoring long-term outcome of stroke and is often used as an indicator of discharge placement after rehabilitation in the elderly unit, as it gives a reasonable indication of the amount of time and assistance the patient requires. However, no physiotherapist would use this index to measure short-term improvements in function as the scaling is too gross. One of the activities measured by the Barthel is ability to transfer. The patient scores 2 if he or she requires minor help (verbal or physical). A patient could improve substantially and yet still score 2. In this instance a more sensitive or responsive outcome measure would be appropriate.

Anatomy of an outcome measure

Outcomes can be good, bad or indifferent. We have all treated patients who have failed to improve or even got worse. The way physiotherapists have traditionally assessed outcome is by comparing the initial assessment with the end assessment, as illustrated in Figure 11.1:

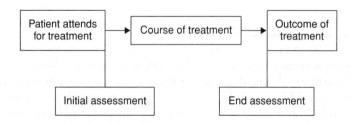

Outcome = End assessment *minus* initial assessment

Figure 11.1   The way physiotherapists have traditionally assessed outcome

If the equation calculates a positive result then the outcome is probably good.

If the equation calculates a negative result then the outcome is probably bad.

If the equation calculates an equal result, then the outcome is probably bad.

For example, pain may be used as an outcome measure in the treatment of a patient with arthritic hips. Classically, pain is measured at initial assessment and the treating physiotherapist notes pain levels at each treatment session. The outcome of treatment is then noted as the pain levels at the end assessment minus the pain levels at the initial assessment. Reduction in pain over the treatment period is deemed to be a positive outcome. However, if the pain has got worse, this is seen as a bad outcome. Similarly, if the pain levels remain unchanged this cannot be seen as a good outcome as the aim of treatment was to reduce the pain, which it clearly has not. This example also shows the importance of using more than one key outcome measure, as the overall outcome of treatment in this case is dependent on several factors. For example, although pain levels might not have changed, other positive outcomes may have been achieved in functional ability and coping strategies.

Outcomes are noted and recorded. There are many measurements already noted in assessments that may be used as outcome measures:

- Objective clinical measurements such as range of movement, swelling
- Subjective clinical measurements such as estimation of range, pallor
- Self-reported measures such as 'better', 'worse', 'the same'
- Pain
- Symptom presentation such as extent of sciatic nerve signs
- Functional ability
- Achievement of goals
- Muscle strength
- Level of fitness/stamina/endurance
- Levels of medication such as for pain, spasticity
- Level of patient knowledge/understanding of their condition
- Use of mobility aids
- Adherence to home programmes.

Could it? Should it? Would it?

Any of these measures may be used as outcome measures. When setting up an audit and involving all participants, it is vital to agree which outcome measures should be used, how they are to be recorded (in a prospective audit) and whether the most appropriate outcome is being used. If in doubt, consider the 'Could it? Should it? Would it?' rule:

Could this outcome measure be used for this population with this condition? Is it valid and responsive enough for use in this particular audit?

Should it be used at all? Is it reliable enough to be used under these circumstances? How could we make it more reliable?

Would this particular choice of outcome measure be appropriate to use? Will it be possible to use this measure across the whole episode of care?

Pre-existing validated health scales

There are many hundreds of health scales being used to measure outcome in research, clinical situations, levels of patient satisfaction and audit. There are scales for almost every eventuality, ranging from the widely used and well recognized, such as the Nottingham Health Profile, to the condition-specific and less well known such as the Varicose Veins Questionnaire. As previously noted, many of these scales are identified and discussed in terms of their validity, reliability and responsiveness in books by Bowling (1991, 1995) and McDowell and Newell (1996). Cole *et al.* (1995) and Wade (1992) look at a number of health measurement scales from a particular physiotherapy stance.

Pre-existing health measurement scales are often more valuable for management or research purposes. It is virtually impossible to find a scale that can suit the purposes of both management for service provision reasons and physiotherapeutic intervention for clinical effectiveness purposes.

The types of measures most commonly used are the following:

- Multi-dimensional profiles, e.g. Medical Outcomes Survey Short Form 36 (SF-36)
- Functional status, e.g. Barthel Index
- Mental health, e.g. Hospital Anxiety and Depression Scale
- Disease specific, e.g. Clinical Back Pain Questionnaire
- Measure of pain, e.g. McGill Pain Questionnaire
- Quality of life, e.g. General Well-Being Schedule
- Social networks and support, e.g. Family Relationship Index
- Patient satisfaction.

The advantages of using health measurement scales are that they are well researched and have a competent track record of use. Many are also robust in terms of inter-rater reliability, i.e. different raters measuring the same person would score the same response. They are excellent to use as outcome measures where very accurate information is needed, such as in research. It is also possible to use them in a multi-centre project, where agreeing on or designing specific outcome measures might be difficult. The disadvantage to many health measurement scales is that they are time-consuming to complete, some require training and some may only be used under licence, adding cost implications to your project.

'Off the shelf' health measurement scales may not completely address your information needs: either a scale may gather too much information, some of which may not be necessary, or it might miss out a question that is crucial to your study. Adding to or removing parts of a validated health measurement scale immediately diminishes its tested validity and may infringe copyright. Sometimes, it is necessary to use several health measurement scales to get the information you seek – adding to data collection time. In a busy physiotherapy department, it is often not practical to use health measurement scales in clinical audit for these reasons. However, it is worth considering the use of health measurement scales as there may well be one that actually suits you very well.

When using health measurement scales, always check to see if any licence or special training is required prior to use. Do not assume that, just because a scale has been published in full, it may be freely used. Always check conditions of copyright, or contact the author of the scale for permission to use it.

Physiotherapy-specific and home-grown outcome measures: some points to remember

Sometimes, it is not appropriate or possible to use pre-existing outcome measures and, in these situations, it is necessary to design your own. It is important to remember that any such measures should be tested for validity and reliability in the situation in which they are to be used. Such measures will not necessarily be appropriate for use in other situations with different populations.

Ensure that the outcome measures actually relate to the standard. Chapter 7 stresses the importance of ensuring the accuracy of any standards you set by basing them on professional knowledge and clinical experience, and backing them up with a literature search to ensure that you are not 're-inventing the wheel' or missing out on important up-to-date research. You may have a standard for the treatment of patients with low back pain which states: 'Patients referred with low back pain will be assessed by a physiotherapist, treated as appropriate to relieve pain, increase range of movement and optimize function to enable them to return to daily activities. Patients will receive education and advice regarding their condition together with a home management programme.'

In order to relate to the standard, the outcome measures need to include:

- Changes in pain level
- Alterations in range of movement
- Changes in function.

You may also want to measure the patient's knowledge of the education and advice you have given. This could be measured simply by testing recall of the last treatment session. Similarly, you could measure adherence to the home exercise programme, although this would depend on how honestly the patient answered your questions.

You may wish to look at outcome of low back pain over time. Rather than recall all of the patients 1 year later and reassess them, it would be easier to telephone them or to send a simple questionnaire that the patients can answer. In order to match the assessments accurately, the outcome measures need to be exactly the same. Therefore, it is of little use having numeric data measured by the physiotherapist in the first assessment and self-reported information from the patient in the second. It does not matter which outcome measures you use so long as they reflect the standard and are repeatable in all the circumstances you wish to apply them. There is considerable value in considering all the options at the outset of an audit to ensure that the correct data are collected in the most appropriate format.

Outcome measures from differing perspectives

An outcome could never be described as 'cut and dried'. The same outcome may mean different things to different people. For example, when you go out to buy new clothes, various outcomes may result. Say, your trip is successful and you purchase exactly what you were after. The outcomes for you are as follows:

- Pleasure with your purchase (good outcome)
- Reduced bank balance (outcome dependent on your financial status)
- Knowledge of which shops suit your requirements (good outcome).

If, however, you fail to purchase anything, your outcomes are as follows:

- Annoyance at nothing purchased (bad outcome)
- Bank balance unaffected (good outcome)
- Knowledge of which shops do not suit your requirements (good outcome).

It can be seen that both these scenarios have mixed outcomes. However, the overriding influence is whether or not you achieved your primary aim – to buy some new clothes. Similarly, we have all treated patients who have made a good recovery but remain totally dissatisfied because they have not achieved their main aim. It is important to use outcome measures that mean something to the therapist, the patient and, where appropriate, the carer, in order to show the effect of physiotherapy intervention.

Agreeing the most appropriate and achievable outcome measures can be difficult if the physiotherapist and patient disagree. When patient and therapist have different perspectives, there is nothing to prevent you from noting both.

Quantity, quality, patient satisfaction, alteration in pathology

The bottom line with outcomes is to identify whether the physiotherapy intervention allows the patient to go further, perform better, feel that the intervention has helped, or to see some improvement in the pathology. It therefore makes sense to measure outcomes in four main areas:

1. Quantity
2. Quality

3. Patient satisfaction or quality of life
4. Alteration in pathology.

Outcomes can have qualitative and quantitative elements. Useful outcome measures for a child with cerebral palsy may relate to the distance and quality of gait. Distance can be measured quantitatively in yards or metres although it may also be appropriate to note the surface, as this can have some bearing on the distance walked. Qualitatively, the gait may be analysed subjectively for cadence, balance and heel strike, either by watching the child as he walks or by analysing a video recording later. Analysis of gait in a gait laboratory allows the qualitative elements of gait to be quantified, but this facility is unlikely to be available readily in standard community paediatric practice. Other qualitative measurements can include subjective impression of smoothness of movement, comfort, alertness, cyanosis and well being.

Quantity does not just have to relate to distance. It can relate to anything with a numeric value including joint range, pain measured on a visual analogue scale or vital capacity. In isolation, a goniometric reading tells us nothing about the outcome of intervention. It is the changes in the reading over the period of treatment that reflect the outcome. Thus, 'an improvement of 30 degrees knee flexion' tells you more than 'knee flexion 110 degrees' and is therefore a useful outcome measure. For a particular patient, a single improvement obtained from before-and-after measurements cannot be defended against the argument that the improvement might have occurred spontaneously. However, this is not a problem with a group of patients where non-intervention is known to produce no improvement in symptoms.

Patient satisfaction is the key to a positive outcome. The main aim of a stroke patient is to walk, but when the physiotherapist has facilitated this through weeks of treatment, the patient may remain dissatisfied, as 'walking' to him or her means tramping across the moors with the dogs, not walking across the gym with a stick! However, careful clarification of 'walking' as an outcome measure in this example could evoke patient satisfaction even if it were still far from the patient's goal. Patient satisfaction surveys are common as part of implementation by trusts of *The Patient's Charter*, and as part of information gathering by purchasers. As part of outcome audit, it may be more appropriate to use quality of life measurement scales. However, use of such scales may be of greater value to managers than to individual clinicians seeking to identify the effectiveness of their interventions – as the outcome indicators or criteria may be too gross to be of much clinical value.

Alteration in pathology can often be an indicator of improvement, e.g. as sciatica diminishes, the pain retreats up the back of the leg. This can be noted and used as an outcome, measuring improvement, and of value to the physiotherapist seeking to measure clinical effectiveness. Similarly, chest X-rays show when infection and sputum retention are reducing and indicate that the patient is getting over a chest infection. In some pathologies, physiotherapy aims to delay the inevitable deterioration.

Boys with muscular dystrophy have a progressive disease but outcome measures such as maintenance of muscle length and walking ability can show the impact (and hopefully, effectiveness) of physiotherapy in the short term. Outcome audit for progressive pathologies can be addressed by using small goal achievement and checklists as described below.

Using goal achievement as an outcome measure

One of the reasons for using outcomes is so that the quality, efficiency and effectiveness of a service can be determined. Data collected during outcome audits can be used successfully in contract negotiation as well as in service evaluation. It is important to be able to provide data that exhibits clinical effectiveness. Physiotherapy managers need to be able to say that the service is reaching its standards for facilitating patient recovery.

How can physiotherapists measure sensitively the improvements of individual patients, whilst providing robust evidence that groups of patients with the same presentations are benefiting from physiotherapy intervention? This is complicated by the fact that all patients react differently, and no two patients ever exhibit exactly the same symptoms or pattern of recovery. It is almost impossible to compare individual patients. It may be fairly easy to predict the course of treatment and recovery time for a patient with an uncomplicated Colles fracture, but virtually impossible for someone with a profound head injury. For people who were fit before their injury or illness, it is possible to identify a prior level of competency for which to aim but, for people with conditions present from birth, there is no such baseline. People with deteriorating pathology cannot make and sustain vast physical improvements by nature of their condition. However, we still need outcome measures that are able to take these factors into account and show that physiotherapy intervention is effective. In this case, group data needed for contracting purposes are readily available by aggregating the results of individuals appropriately.

If we return to our original assumption that patients attend for physiotherapy in order to address a physical problem, then we can use goal achievement as an outcome measure (Barnard, 1995). Although goals themselves differ widely in their number and difficulty, if they are jointly set by the therapist and patient, they will have a degree of validity and appropriateness. It hardly matters that the goals are wide-ranging if successful intervention is measured by the achievement of joint set goals. Joint set goals imply that the outcomes are of value to the patient. A middle-aged woman having treatment following a fractured ankle may be happy to set a goal of pain-free ankle movement whilst driving, with the swelling reduced such that she can wear her normal shoes. A young athlete with exactly the same injury may well require a pain-free ankle whilst running and a greater degree of joint flexibility, and would therefore not value an outcome of the same degree as the woman.

Goal achievement is an outcome measure that can be used in all areas of physiotherapy. Recently, it has been widely used as an outcome measurement by physiotherapists in learning disabilities (Standing, 1997). It can be looked at in terms of the World Health Organization classification of impairment, handicap and disability (Cole *et al.*, 1995). Short-term goals are considered in terms of impairment, medium-term goals in terms of disability, and long-term goals in terms of handicap.

For example, an adult with profound learning and physical disability may have the following goal-orientated programme:

Impairment: Reduce lower limb spasticity; train sitting balance reactions
Disability: Sit on the edge of the bed
Handicap: Become less dependent in dressing.

There is no reason why this model could not be used in other areas, e.g. for an elderly woman with arthritic knees attending a day hospital:

Impairment: Reduce pain and swelling; increase range of movement
Disability: Improve gait and walking distance
Handicap: Go shopping on the bus.

Checklists

There is more to a satisfactory outcome than just a clinical improvement. Physiotherapy includes giving advice, educating patients in their condition, and providing information about other services. We may spend more time with carers than with the actual patient whilst setting up management and maintenance programmes. Physiotherapists working in acute outpatient departments find it relatively easy to show good outcomes to their intervention. Patients leave with decreased pain, increased range of movement and improved function. A community physiotherapist working with patients with deteriorating conditions does not have such an easy task. It is possible to use adherence to home programme as an outcome measure, and carer implementation of lifting and handling regimes. Use checklists relating to the standard (e.g. information given regarding positioning, skin care, assistance with clearing chest secretions, etc.), a good outcome being the satisfactory imparting of that information. It is debatable whether reduced numbers of pressure sores, or lack of increase in joint contracture can also be used as outcome measures. Donabedian (1988) states that patient satisfaction may be one of the desirable outcomes of care and this may be the key outcome measure in some situations.

The following is an example of a checklist used to describe outcome measures for a patient with motor neurone disease (MND) living at home:

- Correct positioning routine taught and
  implemented: Checked yes/no
- Maintenance programme for chest care
  implemented: Checked yes/no
- Patient and carer provided with MND Society
  contact number   Checked yes/no
- Referral to speech and language therapist re:
  swallowing: Checked yes/no.

TELER®

TELER® is the acronym for treatment evaluation by le Roux's method (le Roux, 1993). Originally devised for physiotherapy evaluation, it is now widely used in many rehabilitation services and nursing. The TELER® concept is based on the routine collection of information that is simple, flexible, effective and patient specific. It also presents records in such a way as to show clinical effectiveness, attribution of what happens to the patient who is receiving treatment, and in a layout that can easily be used in clinical audit. The TELER® system is more than just a means of conducting outcome audit. It is a whole patient record keeping system which can be adapted to fulfil legal medical record keeping and identify the progression of treatment. It may also be used in structure and process audit. TELER® is copyright and trade marked, its implementation requires training and the system may only be used under licence. Details of courses and the full extent of the TELER® system are available from TELER®, PO Box 699, Sheffield S17 3YG.

In the TELER® system, outcome is measured using TELER® indicators. There are three types of TELER® indicator. One of these types comprises function indicators which can be useful indicators of outcome in physiotherapy. These are six-point ordinal scales where 0 indicates the deficit that needs to be addressed through treatment and 5 indicates that this deficit has been fully rectified. The points in between are clinically relevant changes that need to be achieved in ascending order before the desired outcome (usually maximal improvement or full function) has been reached (le Roux, 1997). The TELER® indicator is a six-point scale because six points trace five improvements, which are the minimum number needed to demonstrate that a patient who achieves the outcome denoted by point 5 on the scale could not and would not have done so spontaneously (le Roux, private correspondence). The achievement of the goal is therefore attributable to the intervention. Although the TELER® indicator does not identify what that intervention is, a properly completed TELER® form frequently will.

An example of an indicator is 'dynamic sitting' TELER®:

0 Unable to move in sitting
1 Able to move arm
2 Able to anterior and posterior tilt pelvis
3 Able to transfer weight to R and L and return to mid line
4 Able to move leg
5 Able to transfer weight to L and R and rotate to mid line.

The numbers are not scores but codes simply to denote where the patient is in terms of functional ability. As the patient improves (or gets worse) changes are noted in his or her code. It can be seen that once the appropriate indicator has been chosen, it is a simple task just to note the patient's code rather than write out his capabilities and disabilities in full.

It is almost always appropriate to use several indicators, choosing the most relevant for individual patients. It is possible to write specific indicators for individual patients or for specific functional problems. The Bassetlaw POEM (Patient Orientated Evaluation Method) catalogue of indicators (Allerton *et al.*, 1992) (which is also copyright) comprises some 60 six-point indicators that can be used in conjunction with the TELER® system. Some of these indicators may be made patient specific by allowing the patient to identify his or her key problem and relating that to the indicator.

For example, the Bassetlaw POEM indicator P1.1© is as follows:

0 Has pain at all times
1 Pain prevents .... but can do other things
2 Pain interrupts .... and cannot resume
3 Pain interrupts .... but can resume
4 Pain during .... but can do the activity without interruption
5 Pain-free activity.

Once it has been established that the patient complains of an activity that causes pain, it is a simple task to insert the relevant activity for that specific patient. It can be seen that this indicator would be valid for any patient who reports an activity limited by pain. It does not matter where the pain is or what activity causes it, because you can adapt the indicator to fit the patient. Therefore, this indicator could be used for a young man with a sports injury causing shoulder pain that limits him on the squash court or an elderly woman learning to dress again after an operation to repair a fractured hip.

Improvement can be shown graphically by plotting the number of indicators achieved against the number of treatments (Mawson and McCreadie, 1993). Using formulae known as the 'TELER® Index', it is possible to calculate health gain. These formulae are part of the TELER® concept and are available to licence holders.

According to le Roux:

> It is impossible to overstate the importance of emphasizing two crucial facts about TELER. The first is that TELER is a system of clinical note making and the TELER indicator is part of that system. The second is that the TELER indicator is quite unlike the other measuring scales available to clinicians. These other measuring scales are designed to provide clinical information for managers, that is clinical information about groups of patients, and they are designed to measure absolutes, for example, the level of deficit. In contrast, the TELER indicator is designed to provide clinical information for clinicians, that is, clinical information about individual patients, and is designed to trace clinically significant change, for example, clinically significant improvement or deterioration in ability to perform an activities of daily living (ADL) activity.

> (le Roux, personal correspondence)

Examples of actual physiotherapy audits using the TELER® and other approaches are shown in the next chapter.

References

Allerton R., Childs J., Greco M., Jater M. (1992). *Bassetlaw Patient Orientated Evaluation Method*. Bassetlaw Hospital and Community Services NHS Trust, Worksop.

Barnard S. (1993). Outcomes in physiotherapy intervention audit. *Physiotherapy*, **79**, 766.

Barnard S. (1995). Wessex Region Physiotherapy Intervention Audit Project: Models for intervention audit. *Physiotherapy*, **81**, 202–207.

Bowling A. (1991). *Measuring Health: A Review of Quality of Life Measurement Scales*. Open University Press, Milton Keynes.

Bowling A. (1995). *Measuring Disease*. Open University Press, Milton Keynes.

Chartered Society of Physiotherapy (1995). *Outcomes Pack*. 14 Bedford Row, London WC1R 4ED.

Cole B., Finch E., Gowland C., Mayo N. (1995). *Physical Rehabilitation Outcome Measures*. Health Canada and the Canadian Physiotherapy Association, Toronto.

DePoy E., Gitlin L.N. (1993). *Introduction to Research: Multiple Strategies for Health and Human Services*. Mosby, St. Louis.

Donabedian A. (1988). The quality of care: how can it be assessed? *Journal of the American Medical Association*, **260**, 1743–1748.

le Roux A.A. (1993). TELER®: the concept. *Physiotherapy*, **79**, 755–758.

le Roux A.A. (1997). *TELER Information Pack*, 4th edn. TELER®, PO Box 699, Sheffield S17 3YG.

Long A. F. (1994). *Exploring Outcomes in Routine Clinical Practice: A Step-by-Step Guide*. Outcomes Briefing, April 4–9. UK Clearing House for Information on the Assessment of Health Outcomes. The Nuffield Institute for Health, Clarenden Road, Leeds LS2 9PL.

Mawson S., McCreadie M. (1993). TELER®: the way forward in clinical audit. *Physiotherapy*, **79**, 758–761.

McDowell I., Newell C. (1996). *Measuring Health: A Guide to Rating Scales and Questionnaires*, 2nd edn. Oxford University Press.

New South Wales Department of Health (1992). The NSW Health Outcomes Programme. *New South Wales Public Health Bulletin*, **3**, 125.

Outcomes Briefing (1993). Spring issue. UK Clearing House for Information on the Assessment of Health Outcomes. The Nuffield Institute for Health, Clarenden Road, Leeds LS2 9PL.

Standing S. (1997). *Magical, Mythical, Measurable: A Study Of Outcome Measures Used by Physiotherapists in Learning Disabilities*. MSc dissertation. Department of Psychology, University of Portsmouth.

Wade D. (1992). *Measurement in Neurological Rehabilitation*. Oxford University Press.

Whitehead M. (1988). The Health Divide. In *Inequalities in Health*. Penguin, Middlesex.

12
Outcome audit in physiotherapy

The principles of outcome audit, discussed in the previous chapter, are put into practice here. Mawson and McCreadie (1993) identify five existing audit tools to look at outcome:

- Patient satisfaction surveys
- Peer review
- Disease specific measures, e.g. Arthritis Impact Scale
- Topic specific measures, e.g. Barthel Index
- Multi-dimensional health profiles, e.g. Nottingham Health Profile.

We have already noted that the Chartered Society of Physiotherapy recommends the use of pre-existing health measurement scales where possible, as many are claimed to be already validated, and many of the problems with application or analysis have already been ironed out. Many of these scales are entirely appropriate for use in audits to gather gross data about groups of patients. However, it may be necessary to add another tool to the list where there is no appropriate existing scale: home-grown outcome measures.

The type of tool you use will depend upon why you are gathering outcome data. There are different reasons for conducting outcome audits:

- Commissioners may need information about patient throughput, patient satisfaction with your service, and broad-based outcome information such as return to work and re-referral rates for the same condition. This information informs purchasers and potential purchasers about the efficiency and effectiveness of your department and the quality of your service from the patient's perspective.
- Senior physiotherapists may conduct an intervention audit within their team to identify the outcomes of treatment for patients with specific conditions. Sensitive measures are used and the results of the audit analysed to identify any shortfall in expected outcome. The clinical effectiveness of a team or individual may be ascertained in this way by peer review.
- Physiotherapists want to ensure that their patients' treatment is delivered as effectively as possible.

This chapter looks at the practicalities of setting up and running outcome audit – for managerial purposes including contract negotiation with commissioners, from the point of view of patient satisfaction, and for peer review of clinical effectiveness within a team.

Outcome audits are conducted in the same way as any other. Actual practice is audited against agreed, set standards. Defining the standards for outcome audit depends upon the reason for the audit.

Setting standards for outcome audits

It was stated in the previous chapter that outcome audit differs slightly from structure and process audits by virtue of the fact that basing standards and outcome measures on the clinical literature, and up-to-date research findings, is crucial. Outcome standards are based on research findings and clinical experience. They should not be based on clinical experience alone, as you may set standards that are out of line with other clinicians, and this may not be in the best interests of your patients. This is not to say that clinical experience should never be incorporated. Often, physiotherapy interventions have been researched in different environments, or with a different subject group to that of your local setting. Then, it may be necessary to adapt research-based standards and outcomes to your particular service. As more clinical guidelines are incorporated into practice, it will be possible to use these as the standards against which to audit the outcome of intervention. Nationally agreed guidelines, such as those formulated by the Royal College of General Practitioners, the Chartered Society of Physiotherapy, the Osteopathic Association of Great Britain, the British Chiropractic Association, and the National Back Pain Association, for the management of acute low back pain (Waddell *et al.*, 1996), lend themselves to division into measurable criteria which can be audited. Where these well-researched and agreed guidelines exist, it is recommended that they are used in both service delivery and evaluation. The National Health Service Executive states that: 'The Clinical Outcomes Group has recommended that, while all the guidelines it endorses are acceptable aids to clinical practice, only those based on evidence from RCTs (randomized controlled trials) should be used in contract specification.' (NHSE, 1996)

As yet, relatively little physiotherapy intervention has been subjected to randomized controlled trials or other robust methodologies, although it is possible to access up-to-date research findings, from the literature, as previously discussed. Some national physiotherapy clinical guidelines now exist and these can be used as a basis for outcome audits in the same way as the professional standards (CSP, 1993) can be used in structure and process audits.

Identifying research findings from the literature

The professional body is a good source of up-to-date knowledge and will conduct literature searches for a small fee. The following references of review articles on physiotherapy effectiveness are currently available from the Chartered Society of Physiotherapy and are added to and updated on a regular basis (CSP, 1996a–g):

- Back pain
- Cardiopulmonary rehabilitation
- Electrophysical agents
- Incontinence
- Neurology
- Orthopaedics and rheumatology
- Paediatrics.

Other sources available in medical libraries are database literature searches such as Medline, Bids, Cinahl, etc. *Effective Health Care* bulletins and *Effectiveness Matters* publications are available from the NHS Centre for Reviews and Dissemination at the University of York. The Cochrane collaboration undertakes systematic reviews and these are available on CD ROM or by contacting the Cochrane Centre. The information pack *Clinical Effectiveness Reference Pack*, produced by the NHSE (1996), is a useful source of further information. More recently, the National Centre for Clinical Audit (NCCA) of which the Chartered Society of Physio-therapy is a founder partner, offers a wide range of literature search facili-ties and clinical audit project models, which can be accessed, in the first instance, by contacting the Professional Affairs Department of the CSP. It is also worth mentioning here that one of the functions of trust clinical audit departments is to provide 'audit library' facilities, and it may be possible to access many of the above-mentioned resources, on-site, by contacting the audit department.

Outcome audit for commissioners

As with any audit, it is important to define clearly the reasons for con-ducting the project, and to involve everyone who has a stake in the ser-vice or intervention being audited. Purchasers and prospective purchasers will need broad-based outcomes to give them an overview of the service. They may insist upon specific outcome measures so that they can compare your service with others (benchmarking). Almost certainly, they will not be interested in very fine measures of physiotherapy intervention of the kind used by therapists in patient assessment, to ascertain recovery or clin-ical effectiveness, such as range of movement, amount of swelling, etc. They are more likely to require broad-based physiotherapy outcomes such as return to work or overall recovery. Similarly, purchasers buying surgical operations are more interested in mortality rates, length of hospital stay and percentages of wound infection, rather than specific information about the minutiae of the operation and subsequent recovery. While the latter information is vital to surgeons seeking to improve their techniques, it has less relevance to purchasers who need to make informed decisions about purchasing surgery for a local health population.

Outcome audits for commissioners can be used in three different ways:

- As evidence to tender for contracts for physiotherapy services
- As evaluation of services already being purchased
- As evidence to bid for extra funding for new resources, e.g. staff, equipment, etc.

Evidence for tendering

Gathering outcome audit information from existing services is important for a department which intends to tender for new contracts. For example, an established hospital physiotherapy department may wish to tender for contracts with local fundholding general practitioners. The GPs will have a good idea about the services they require, and the physiotherapy managers will have a good idea about the service they can offer. Much discussion will centre around the structure and process issues of cost and service delivery, but the measurable health outcome of physiotherapy intervention is the key to the contract being placed – this, after all, is why the GPs wish to purchase physiotherapy services in the first place! An audit of existing outcomes in a local unit will tell you how soon patients are discharged due to resolution of their condition or problem, and how many re-attend because of recurrence of that condition. This information is also useful when negotiating the length of time required for treating patients, i.e. until the majority of their symptoms resolve, or until they achieve joint set goals and can continue their recovery with a home programme.

Evaluation of current service

When a service is purchased, standards of outcome need to be agreed between physiotherapists and purchasers to ensure that respective expectations are the same. An audit of these outcome standards, once a service contract has commenced, informs both the purchaser and the provider of the service of any shortfall in the system which may need to be addressed – either through increased efficiency, by more stringent adherence to referral guidelines, or provision of alternative resources.

Evidence of need

All services are continually developing and, with them, the need for flexibility in service delivery and provision. Contracts are usually agreed for a set period. During this time, circumstances may change, i.e. there may be an unexpected increase in the patient load, or deficiencies may be identified in the original contract, e.g. a particular patient group may have been mistakenly omitted from the initial calculations. The physiotherapy service may notice a shortfall in resources and undertake an outcome audit

Table 12.1   Example of outcome audit

Aim: To evaluate the effectiveness of treatment of acute ankle sprain

Patient population

Age 16–40 years
Male and female
Injury within 2 weeks of referral
Referred via A & E or GP.

Exclusions

Rupture of ligaments
Fractures.

Standard
Patients will improve substantially and be ready for discharge within 3 weeks of initial contract.

Threshold compliance: 95%

Criteria for discharge (outcome measures):

1. Stand on affected leg for 1 minute without support
2. Range of movement = 75% of inversion of affected ankle when compared to unaffected ankle
3. Hop on affected leg × 10 without support
4. Treadmill on lowest resistance/speed for 5 minutes
5. Discharge within 3 weeks of first attendance.

Results
94 patients attended with this diagnosis over a 2-year period.
19 excluded: failed to meet criteria/ DNA*/specific outcome measures not tested/recorded in notes.

Of 75 patients included in the audit:

89.4% met all criteria
10.6% met all criteria except discharge within 3 weeks.

Total treatments: 254
Average course of treatment: 3.4 attendances
Average episode of care: 9 days.

Action

1. Discuss findings with outpatient staff
2. Promote as an example of cost-effective treatment with purchasers and potential purchasers
3. Threshold for compliance should be reduced to 90%
4. Look into reason for 10% failure rate.

Re-audit in 1 year.

(Reproduced with permission.)
*DNA, did not attend.

to add weight to its request for additional resources. Robust data will improve your basis for renewed negotiation.

Table 12.1 shows an example of outcome audit (reproduced with permission) to evaluate the effectiveness of the treatment of acute ankle sprain. This audit clarifies for purchasers whether their agreed set standard is being achieved.

Patient satisfaction outcome audits

Patient satisfaction surveys are becoming common in health service management. Health authorities are required to ascertain the healthcare needs of their populations, and to ensure that these are being met. Commissioners often carry out their own surveys to measure patient satisfaction with the services being purchased on their behalf. NHS trust managers may conduct patient satisfaction surveys to see if they are reaching *Patient's Charter* targets. Physiotherapy departments are likely to survey patients to identify whether standards are being reached, from the patient's perspective, in order to improve or develop services.

The theory behind writing patient satisfaction questionnaires is discussed in Chapters 3 and 6, and issues of consumer involvement in audit in Chapter 15.

Table 12.2 demonstrates an audit of patient satisfaction undertaken amongst women attending a continence clinic. The service had been running for 5 years and the physiotherapy manager wanted a full evaluation of the service as there was purchaser interest in expanding the service to other areas of the trust.

The survey provided valuable information for both the service providers and purchasers. However, several factors need to be taken into consideration. Firstly, the survey response rate was 55% and, although this is reasonable for a postal survey, there is a possibility that non-respondents failed to reply due to dissatisfaction or embarrassment. However, it could also be interpreted that these women had the opportunity to express their opinions and chose to decline. Secondly, the standards are written in the non-assertive format 'should'. Standards are a statement of intent and should be written in the more assertive 'will' format to identify clearly the expectations.

Outcome audits for clinical effectiveness

Outcome audits are becoming more important now that there is a greater emphasis on clinical effectiveness and evidence-based practice. Outcome audits are a means of checking actual outcomes of physiotherapy intervention against expected outcomes identified by research, clinical guidelines and professional standards.

The example illustrated in Tables 12.3–12.5 (reproduced with permission) shows some of the key elements of an outcome audit that investigates

Table 12.2 Physiotherapy continence clinic audit – patient satisfaction

Patient population
Explanatory letters and questionnaires issued to all patients attending the continence clinic over a 4-month period.

Exclusions: None.

Standard 1
Patients attending the physiotherapy continence clinic should be satisfied with the service they receive. 90% threshold compliance.

Standard 2
After attending patients should experience a decrease in symptoms.

Criteria for satisfaction

1. Satisfied that initial session was conducted in a group
2. Satisfied with size of the group
3. Satisfied with length of the session
4. Satisfied with age mix of the group
5. Satisfied with waiting time between referral and group session
6. Satisfied with clarity of the information
7. Satisfied with relevance of the information
8. Satisfied with amount of information
9. Satisfied with quality of the handouts
10. Experience an improvement in symptoms since attending the clinic.

Results

28 of the attending 51 patients returned the completed questionnaires.
92.8% of the responding patients were satisfied with the service they received, thus achieving standard 1.
70% of responding patients (19) noted an improvement in symptoms since attending the clinic.
Standard 2 was not met by all attendees.

Action

1. Look into the reasons why standard 2 was not met. Consider changes in practice to raise the threshold.
2. Physiotherapists will continue to offer individual consultations to patients who do not wish to attend group sessions.
3. Standard 2 to be re-written: After attending the initial session patients should experience a decrease in symptoms within 2 months.
4. Undertake a survey across the rest of the trust to identify any continence clinic need in other areas.
5. Re-audit in 2 years.

(Reproduced with permission.)

whether standards regarding home exercise programmes are being achieved. No existing health measurement scale was felt to be appropriate so 'home-grown' outcome measures were agreed by the physiotherapists undertaking the audit. This audit measures patient compliance (outcome) with the home exercise and management regime provided by physiotherapists (process).

Table 12.3   Audit of home exercises: Protocol

Background

Home exercises are an important and integral part of a patient's treatment plan. Lack of patient compliance in this area can lead to treatment being prolonged or, at worst, failure to improve. Home exercises also enable the patients to help themselves and become more self-reliant, thus saving physiotherapy time and increasing the efficiency of the department.

Objective

To identify patients' compliance with home exercise and management regimes.

Subjects

50 consecutive patients of all ages attending outpatient physiotherapy.

Exclusions: None.

Time period: 3 weeks.

(Reproduced with permission.)

Table 12.4   Audit of home exercises: Standards

Standard	Threshold compliance	Exceptions	Definitions and instructions for data retrieval
1. Patients are required to do a home exercise regime	100%	None	Documented in patient orientated medical records (POMR)
2. Patients are instructed on which exercise and number of repetitions	100%	None	Type of exercise and number documented in POMR
3. Patients are asked after 1 week:			
(a) To recall the number of repetitions for each exercise	100%	DNA*	Documented in POMR
(b) If they completed the required number	100%	DNA	Documented in POMR
(c) To demonstrate correctly each home exercise.	100%	DNA	Documented in POMR

(Reproduced with permission.)
*DNA, did not attend.

Table 12.5   Audit of home exercises: Outcome

Results

1. Patients required to do a home exercise: 100% met the standard.
2. Patients instructed on which exercise and number of repetitions: 100% met the standard.
3. Patients asked after 1 week:

(a) To recall the number of repetitions for each exercise
      72% met the standard, no exclusions
      28% failed to meet the standard.
(b) Whether they completed the required number of exercises
      44% met the standard, no exclusions
      56% failed to meet the standard.
(c) To demonstrate correctly each home exercise
      78% met the standard, no exclusions
      22% failed to meet the standard.

These results were discussed at a staff meeting. Only 44% of patients had completed the correct number of exercises despite 72% remembering how many were required. 78% were able to demonstrate their home exercises 1 week after being taught. The physiotherapists were not happy with these results and discussed ways to improve patient compliance with home exercise programmes. A re-audit was agreed once practice changes had been implemented.

Changes in practice

1. Physiotherapists to emphasize more clearly the importance of complying with home exercises and encourage self-reliance.
2. Physiotherapists to spend more time teaching and checking home exercises.
3. Patients to be issued with a compliance form on which they can mark down when they do their exercises, what and how many they do and any inhibiting factors. Patients to be encouraged to bring this sheet to treatment sessions and discuss it with their physiotherapist.

Re-audit
A re-audit was undertaken 6 months later. The original standards remained the same, but two were added relating to the issue and completion of the compliance forms.

Re-audit results

1. Patients required to do a home exercise. 100% met the standard.
2. Patients instructed on which exercise and number of repetitions. 100% met the standard.
3. Patients asked after 1 week:

(a) To recall the number of repetitions for each exercise
      98% met the standard, no exclusions
      2% failed to meet the standard.
(b) If they completed the required number of exercises
      82% met the standard, no exclusions
      18% failed to meet the standard.
(c) To demonstrate correctly each home exercise
      98% met the standard, no exclusions
      2% failed to meet the standard.

Table 12.5 – *contd*

4. Compliance form completed. 100% met the standard.

Conclusion
The results showed an increase in the number of patients remembering and completing their home exercises. Although these results came much closer to achieving the standard of 100% compliance, the physiotherapy department still felt that improvements could be made and considered involving members of the patient's family (where appropriate and agreement given) to give encouragement at home.
   It was agreed to include compliance forms into general usage.

Future audit
A further audit was planned to measure whether the number of treatments has been reduced in those patients using compliance forms.

(Reproduced with permission.)

The initial audit results show that a problem exists. As it stands, it shows that between 22% and 56% of patients fail to meet the set standard. Although this shows the extent of the problem it does not show the severity. To show this, it would be necessary to examine the data more closely to ascertain the percentage who failed to reach all three standards. This percentage is provided by a different method of analysis described in the *TELER Information Pack* (le Roux, 1997). A similar analysis could be conducted on the results of the re-audit.

Outcome audits using TELER®

In the previous chapter we looked at how TELER® may be used to identify clinically and functionally relevant changes during a course of physiotherapy. TELER® indicators and other similar six-point indicators such as Bassetlaw Patient Orientated Evaluation Method (POEM) indicators can be used as measures of outcome in audit. Standards are based on clinical guidelines, clinical experience, or both, and are linked to relevant indicators. Improvement in individual patients and groups of patients may be shown by the number of improvement steps they make over the treatment period. The following example is reproduced with permission.

Outcome audit of an acute low back pain service

Background
This new service had been in operation in 16 GP surgeries for 1 year. The purchasers and clinicians wished to evaluate its impact. Figures relating to uptake and throughput had already been collected together with a patient satisfaction survey. These results looked promising, but it was necessary to see whether the new service was actually being effective. Patient records had been kept, using the TELER® system, based on a pool of eight indica-

tors previously agreed by the physiotherapy team and based on clinical guidelines.

Objective

To conduct a retrospective audit of physiotherapy records of all patients who had passed through the new service in the previous 12 months to identify the effectiveness of the service.

Standards

Four key outcome standards were agreed:

1. There will be an increased range of pain-free movement
2. Functional activities limited by pain will be restored
3. Sleeping patterns affected by acute back pain will be relieved
4. Referred symptoms linked with the acute back pain will be reduced.

Outcome indicators

On examination, the physiotherapist chose the relevant outcome indicators for each individual patient from the list of eight below:

P1.2 Pain range of movement (© *Bassetlaw Hospital & Community Services NHS Trust*)

Choose painful range of movement relevant to individual patient:

0 Has pain at all times
1 No pain at rest but pain produced by all movements
2 Some movements pain free but .... still painful and limited
3 Pain on repeated .... only
4 Pain on end of .... only
5 Pain-free at all times.

P1.1 Pain activites (© *Bassetlaw Hospital & Community Services NHS Trust*)

Choose painful activity relevant to individual patient:

0 Has pain at all times
1 Pain prevents .... but can do other things
2 Pain interrupts .... and can not resume
3 Pain interrupts .... but can resume
4 Pain during .... but can do this activity without interruption
5 Pain-free activity.

S4.1 Sleeping (1) (© *Bassetlaw Hospital & Community Services NHS Trust*)

0 Total disruption of sleep pattern
1 Is unable to adopt usual sleeping position and wakes more than usual
2 Has difficulty getting into usual position and wakes more than usual
3 Has difficulty getting into usual position, does not wake more than usual

    4 Normal sleeping pattern but has problems on waking (please specify)

    5 Normal sleeping pattern, no problems on waking.

S4.2 Sleeping (2) (© *Bassetlaw Hospital & Community Services NHS Trust*)

    0 Total disruption of sleeping pattern

    1 Has sleep disturbed by pain and *unable* to go back to sleep

    2 Has sleep disturbed by pain but *is able* to go back to sleep

    3 Sleep disturbed but pain present on waking in a.m.

    4 Sleep undisturbed but pain present on waking in a.m. but relieved by activity

    5 Has normal sleeping and waking pattern.

G1.1 General purpose sustained activity (© *Bassetlaw Hospital & Community Services NHS Trust*)

Choose painful activity relevant to individual patient:

    0 Has pain at all times

    1 Pain prevents .... but is able to perform some activities without pain

    2 Pain limits .... time

    3 Has pain during and after .... but time not limited

    4 Is able to .... but has pain afterwards

    5 No pain during or after .... however long.

Activities could include: driving, knitting, walking, cleaning windows, etc.

C3.1 Centralization of pain (McKenzie) (© *Bassetlaw Hospital & Community Services NHS Trust*)

    0 Symptoms in back and down leg into foot

    1 Symptoms in back and down leg to below knee but not into foot

    2 Symptoms in back and down leg to above the knee

    3 Symptoms in back and buttock

    4 Central back pain only

    5 Symptom free.

P1.3 Pain relief by ...., e.g. traction, exercises (© *North Notts Acute Back Pain Service*)

    0 Pain relief up to 30 minutes

    1 Pain relief up to 2 hours

    2 Pain relief up to 12 hours

    3 Pain relief up to 24 hours

    4 Pain relief over 24 hours

    5 Pain-free 3+ days.

P1.4 Pain referral (© *North Notts Acute Back Pain Service*)

    0 Pain referred to lower legs

    1 Pain referred to lower thighs

    2 Pain referred to buttocks

3 Pain centralizing but not maintained
4 Pain abolished but not maintained
5 Pain-free.

The audit

Each set of patient records was checked to see how many patients had achieved improvement in their chosen indicators. Health gain for individual patients and the entire cohort was calculated using the TELER® index (further information about the TELER® system and licensing details are available from A.A. le Roux, TELER, PO Box 699, Sheffield S17 3YG).

Results

Results of the audit showed that 81% of patients using this service had improved by more than 60% from initial assessment; 59% improved by more than 90%. The average health gain for all patients using the service was 78%. (Used with permission: Margaret Jater, Physiotherapy Manager, Bassetlaw Hospital & Community Services NHS Trust.)

The above outcome audit fulfils two roles. Firstly, it shows purchasers that the service is effective and that the contract is worth renewing. Secondly, it informs clinicians that their intervention is clinically effective and that they are achieving their standards. A meeting of all the physiotherapists involved in the service could revisit the standards and indicators to see if these were adequately addressing the activity and functional needs of the patients.

Choice of the most appropriate indicators is absolutely crucial. A patient presenting with pain and limitation of movement should have indicators that reflect both. Otherwise, if only an indicator for pain is used, it may seem from the records that the patient has fully recovered when, in effect, only the pain has improved and range remains static. In order to be truly indicative of outcome of treatment, this system requires both physiotherapist and patient to agree those indicators which reflect each of the patient's presenting problems.

Setting up an outcome audit – Summary

Setting up an outcome audit is no different from setting up any other audit – the practical details can be found in Chapter 7. However, the following brief summary recaps the key requirements:

1. Identify what you need to audit (see Chapter 7)
2. Identify for whom you are doing the audit and design it accordingly
3. Involve all parties who have an interest
4. Identify any pre-existing standards and clinical guidelines
5. Conduct a literature review and use research findings to inform any new standards
6. Agree and set standards, specific outcome measures and percentage thresholds for compliance
7. Agree a project co-ordinator

8. Design the project:

   What timescale?
   Which departments?
   Which patient group, any exclusions?
   Who collects the data?
   Concurrent or retrospective?
   Create and pilot data collection sheet

9. Conduct the audit
10. Discuss results with all involved parties
11. Implement any necessary changes in practice necessary to achieve standards
12. Re-audit to evaluate impact of changes.

References

Chartered Society of Physiotherapy (1993). *Standards of Physiotherapy Practice*, 2nd edn. 14 Bedford Row, London W1R 4ED.

Chartered Society of Physiotherapy (1996a). *References of Review Articles on Physiotherapy Effectiveness: Back Pain*. 14 Bedford Row, London WC1R 4ED.

Chartered Society of Physiotherapy (1996b). *References of Review Articles on Physiotherapy Effectiveness: Cardiopulmonary Rehabilitation*. 14 Bedford Row, London WC1R 4ED.

Chartered Society of Physiotherapy (1996c). *References of Review Articles on Physiotherapy Effectiveness: Electrophysical Agents*. 14 Bedford Row, London WC1R 4ED.

Chartered Society of Physiotherapy (1996d). *References of Review Articles on Physiotherapy Effectiveness: Incontinence*. 14 Bedford Row, London WC1R 4ED.

Chartered Society of Physiotherapy (1996e). *References of Review Articles on Physiotherapy Effectiveness: Neurology*. 14 Bedford Row, London WC1R 4ED.

Chartered Society of Physiotherapy (1996f). *References of Review Articles on Physiotherapy Effectiveness: Orthopaedics and Rheumatology*. 14 Bedford Row, London WC1R 4ED.

Chartered Society of Physiotherapy (1996g). *References of Review Articles on Physiotherapy Effectiveness: Paediatrics*. 14 Bedford Row, London WC1R 4ED.

le Roux A.A. (1997). M1.1 *TELER® for Managers, TELER Information Pack*, 4th edn. TELER, PO Box 699, Sheffield S17 3YG.

Mawson S.J., McCreadie M.J. (1993). TELER, the way forward. *Physiotherapy*, **79**, 758–761.

NHSE (1996). *Clinical Effectiveness Reference Pack*. Crown Copyright. NHSE, Leeds.

Waddell G., Feder G., McIntosh A., Lewis M., Hutchinson A. (1996). *Low Back Pain Evidence Review*. Royal College of General Practitioners, London.

13

Role of the physiotherapist in multiprofessional audit

Physiotherapists are used to working as part of the multiprofessional team on the wards, in rehabilitation units, with paediatrics and the elderly, and in the community. When a patient is receiving medical care and advice from many different clinicians, it is almost impossible to attribute improvement to one particular intervention. It is often more appropriate to audit the impact of the whole multiprofessional service than individual modalities. However, this will always depend upon what is being audited and what the information is going to be used for. For example, a multi-professional process audit will be required if purchasers want information about the efficiency of a stroke unit, but a uniprofessional outcome audit may be more appropriate if, for example, physiotherapists want to check that standards for seating provision are being met in a learning disability service.

The multiprofessional team: audits in parallel

Multiprofessional teams often provide different elements of a complete package of care for the patient. In reality, this often means that patients are receiving several different interventions at once, as illustrated in Figure 13.1.

Many multiprofessional teams work within directorates within the NHS. They often comprise a core of senior, experienced staff used to working together, with regular rotations of junior medical, therapy and nursing staff. An audit undertaken within a multiprofessional team can be described as an evaluation of a service, delivered by a team working in par-allel with each other and the patient. Any form of service evaluation can create or highlight tensions within the team, although working together in multiprofessional audit can also strengthen the team and enhance its attributes.

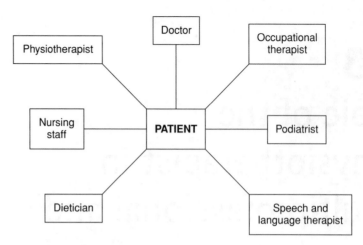

Figure 13.1 Multiprofessional teams provide different elements of a complete package of care for the patient

The term clinical audit may be used to denote both multiprofessional audit in a clinical setting and uniprofessional audit within a clinical setting (Hartigan, 1994).

Multiprofessional audits follow the same pattern as any other audit. They may be structure audits (to optimize facilities and resources, including skill-mix), process audits (to ensure the efficiency of the team especially at the interface of individual professional input), or outcome audit (to see if multiprofessional guidelines, such as those relating to stroke, are being achieved).

Setting up multiprofessional audits

More than ever, in a multiprofessional audit, good communication between team members is vital. This starts at the stage where the decision is made as to what will be audited and continues throughout the process of setting up and running the audit, and includes feedback sessions where possible improvements to practice are discussed and agreed.

Deciding what to audit

This may already have been decided by purchasers who require an evaluation of the service they are purchasing. If you have a free hand in the topic, it is better to brainstorm along the lines suggested in Chapter 7. If the team cannot agree on a single topic, then at least agree to differ and put the other suggestions to one side to be audited next time. Much valuable time can be lost to unnecessary discussion. The final decision must have at least the co-operation, if not the wholehearted agreement, of the entire team. Much is down to the project leader.

Deciding who leads the project

This needs to be someone who has the respect of all the team members and everyone else who will be involved in the audit. It does not need to be the most senior member of the multiprofessional team. It does not even have to be a member of the team. If funding is available for this project from agreed audit monies within a contract, or from another source, the team might consider appointing a clinical audit assistant or officer to manage and undertake the audit. If this is not possible, and so long as the whole team agrees to defer to the audit project leader, it can be a formative experience for a more junior member of the team to take on this responsibility. A Senior II on a longer rotation could gain useful experience towards continuing professional development through this experience.

Leading the project

Having given the project leader the right to lead the audit, the multiprofessional team has implicitly agreed to follow that lead. This is not to say that the project leader has free rein; indeed he or she must continue to liaise with the multiprofessional team, and the multiprofessional team must co-operate with the audit.

Identifying and agreeing standards

The usual principles of setting audit standards apply to multiprofessional audits as to any other. Check what standards are already in place and use them, or develop team standards that are in line with current literature and practice, national and local guidelines. Agreement on multiprofessional standards is key. Where different professions appear to have different standards, agree to use the standards that most accurately reflect the philosophy and practice of your particular team.

Agreeing audit tools

Members of the team may have tried and tested audit tools that they wish to apply to a multiprofessional audit. The team should scrutinize these prior to implementation to check that they are compatible with the whole team's record keeping methods. Pre-existing, validated health measurement scales can be very useful tools for multiprofessional outcome audit, as they often encompass many aspects of the patient's health problems and functional status. Clinical audit officers and assistants are a valuable resource when deciding how to gather data, and it is prudent to take their advice. Agreeing on an audit tool can be very time consuming; it may be helpful to pilot several suggestions on a very small amount of data before finalizing the tool.

Gathering the data

This may be the role of the project leader, members of the multiprofessional team, or an audit assistant. Ensure that everyone who needs to know actually does know who is gathering the data, what information is being gathered and when they are likely to be doing it.

Keeping on track

The project leader has responsibility for keeping the audit on track and on time. Identifying a time scale and a task list in the protocol at the beginning of the project gives a benchmark against which to measure progress. The protocol can be used both as a 'carrot' to speed active participation and as a 'stick' to remind team members of their agreed responsibilities.

Feeding back

This can be an encouraging or a difficult time depending upon the results of the audit. This is the opportunity for the team to review its practice critically in the light of the results, and it should be conducted in an open, blame-free atmosphere.

Effect of clinical audit on the multiprofessional team

If the audit has been conducted thoroughly, with all parties in agreement and good communication maintained throughout, the team will be strengthened by the experience. The information gleaned will enable the team to optimize its practice and maintain or develop high standards of service delivery. Where an audit project exposes strained relations, the feedback session can be used constructively, with diplomatic leadership, to encourage a commitment to better team working. Multiprofessional team audit can be a very useful experience, not only in its primary role to promote service efficiency and effectiveness, but also as a team-building exercise.

Across an episode of care: audits in series

Patients do not always stay within one directorate on their journey through the health system. It is quite common for an elderly person who has had a fall to pass from Accident and Emergency through the orthopaedic directorate to the elderly care unit. It is feasible to audit the interface between directorates to optimize efficiency of handover in order to provide quality of continuing care. This is especially necessary if directorates are on different sites, further limiting easy communication between clinicians. These audits can be seen to occur 'in series'; that is, the care

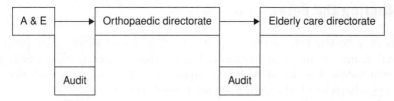

Figure 13.2 Audits occuring at the interface in series

provided by one directorate or department follows on from another, as illustrated in Figure 13.2.

Structure and process audits at the point of handover are probably more pertinent to quality of care than outcome audits at this point.

The same organizational difficulties as with multiprofessional team audits need to be addressed. The main difficulty is that, whilst members of the multiprofessional team know each other well, this may not be the case between directorates, requiring even more scrupulous attention to inter-clinician communication. However, this may not always be the case when auditing the input of one profession between directorates. Despite working within different directorates, physiotherapists are often employed within one department and therefore know one another fairly well. Such a project could be managed by a physiotherapy manager from within the department, again facilitating the process.

Example of multiprofessional audit

Audit of transfer of amputee patients for physiotherapy from surgical directorate to the disablement services centre (DSC) in the rehabilitation directorate.

Background

1. Not all amputee patients are being referred to the DSC from the surgical directorate for physiotherapy.
2. DSC physiotherapists are not seeing all the amputees on the surgical unit prior to transfer to explain the long-term rehabilitation process.

Objective

1. To ensure amputee patients do not slip through the physiotherapy net between directorates.
2. To ensure all amputee patients are aware of the physiotherapy services available within the DSC.

Standards

Standards were agreed after discussion with the two teams of physiotherapists (see Table 13.1). It was decided to implement the standards and audit after 4 months. The aim was to achieve 100% compliance.

Table 13.1 Audit of transfer of amputee patients

Standard	Responsibility	Instructions for data retrieval
1. Name, date of birth, diagnosis and surgical procedure of all lower limb amputees will be passed to the DSC physiotherapy department, in writing, within 3 days of the patient's surgery	Treating ward physiotherapist	Patient information from medical records Referral date noted in physiotherapy records
2. DSC physiotherapists to arrange a suitable time to meet with new amputee patients and treating surgical ward physiotherapist within 3 working days of referral	DSC physiotherapist	Meeting time noted in physiotherapy records
3. Meeting to take place prior to patient being discharged from the ward	DSC physiotherapist	Record of meeting noted in physiotherapy records

The audit

Retrospective process audit. A clinical audit assistant was employed to identify the patients and to trawl through their physiotherapy records for the relevant information.

Subjects

All lower limb amputee patients passing through the surgical directorate over the last 4 months.

Exclusions

Patients living outside the DSC referral area.

Results

The audit was conducted by the audit assistant over a 2-week period, followed by feedback to the physiotherapists concerned. 22 patients passed through the surgical wards for lower limb amputation. Three of those patients lived outside the DSC catchment area and were excluded from the audit.

Standard 1: 75% of patients were referred on to the DSC physiotherapists within 3 days of the patient's surgery. 20% were referred within a week. One patient was not referred at all.

Standard 2: 55% of meetings between the physiotherapists and patient were arranged within 3 working days of receiving the referral.

Standard 3: 95% of patients were visited by the DSC physiotherapists prior to discharge.

Issues arising

The audit improved communications between the two physiotherapy departments by formalizing the referral system. It proved impossible to meet standard 2 at 100% compliance due to the workload and clinical responsibilities within the DSC. The opportunity for patients to fall through the net still existed.

Changes in practice

The clinical audit assistant often found it difficult to obtain exact information from the physiotherapy records to conduct this audit. The record sheet was changed to contain referral boxes so that treating physiotherapists could see at a glance whether a patient had been referred or not.

The DSC physiotherapists set aside regular times for visiting new patients on the surgical wards. The referring physiotherapists then sent the referral to the physiotherapy assistant in the DSC, who booked in a visit and informed both departments and the patient.

It was agreed to retain the 3-day referral timing in standard 2 to see if the changes in practice would enable it to be achieved at the next audit.

Re-audit

The teams agreed to implement the changes in practice and re-audit 6 months later.

Reference

Hartigan G. (1994). Demystifying clinical audit. *Physiotherapy*, **80**, 863–868.

14
Moving towards interface and inter-agency audit

Interface audit

Interface audit describes audit across the interface of different elements of healthcare, for example between primary and secondary care. More and more physiotherapists are now working within primary care, having won contracts with GPs to provide general physiotherapy clinics or specialist services such as back schools. Naturally, both GP and physiotherapist will wish to evaluate the service and the usual structure, process and outcome audits can be undertaken to identify and improve quality, efficiency and effectiveness. There will be times, however, when some patients requiring specialist services need to be referred on from primary care physiotherapists to the hospital department, and vice versa. The efficiency of this interface may be audited by means of an interface audit.

The format of an interface audit is exactly the same as any other, i.e. checking that existing practice meets set standards. It differs only in that it covers two separate departments with different employees. As both may have their own standards and differing codes of practice or guidelines, it is vital that any 'interface standards' are agreed early on. Again, good communication is key to the agreement of standards and the actual audit process.

Setting up an interface audit

- Set standards for resources (structure), service delivery (process) and treatment expectation (outcome) as early as possible, preferably when setting up the contract
- Define and agree an annual audit programme for continuous evaluation in collaboration with colleagues across the interface
- Consult all involved parties (this may include the GPs, practice manager and hospital physiotherapy manager, as well as the physiotherapists working in primary care and the hospital outpatient department)
- Agree well-defined and measurable audit topics

- Identify a project manager
- Design the data collection form and agree who is to collect the data.

Example of an interface audit

Physiotherapists in primary care are referring some patients for hydrotherapy. This is an expensive form of treatment and clinicians working in a fundholding general practice, whose patients are referred, want assurance that the referral process is as efficient as possible.

The audit
A process audit to establish the efficiency of the referral system.

Standards
These were agreed locally between the fundholding GPs and local physiotherapy department when the contract was negotiated:

1. The primary care physiotherapist will assess the patient for suitability for hydrotherapy before any referral is made by the GPs
2. Suitable patients will be told by the primary care physiotherapist whether or not they are to be referred on for hydrotherapy
3. The primary care physiotherapist will send a written referral to the hydrotherapy department within 1 working day of the assessment
4. The physiotherapy assistant in the hydrotherapy department will send a card to the patient detailing his or her appointments (or notification of being put on the waiting list) within 2 working days of receipt
5. The hydrotherapy physiotherapist will send details of attendance and outcome to the referring primary care physiotherapist or GP (as appropriate) within 3 working days of discharge.

Method

- Primary care and hydrotherapy physiotherapists meet to discuss the format of the audit
- Physiotherapists identify all patients referred for hydrotherapy from this practice over the past 6 months from physiotherapy records
- The general practice manager agrees to one of the practice clerical staff pulling all appropriate patient records and checking for standards 1, 2 and 3
- A physiotherapy assistant from the hospital physiotherapy department is asked to check actual practice as noted on the physiotherapy records against standards 4 and 5
- The primary care and hydrotherapy physiotherapist liaise to compile and discuss the full results.

Results
Over the previous 6 months, the therapists identify 12 patients who have been referred for hydrotherapy from the GP practice.

The standards have been met as follows:

Standard 1	100%
Standard 2	100%
Standard 3	91%
Standard 4	33%
Standard 5	50%.

Discussion

From this audit, it became clear that the process was running efficiently from the primary care side but much less efficiently from the hydrotherapy department. The hydrotherapy physiotherapist agreed to look into the reasons why her department was not reaching the standards. She said she would discuss the findings and implications with her manager. The primary care physiotherapist agreed to discuss, with the general practice staff, the possible need to change the standards to make them more workable, although she warned her colleague that it was unlikely that the GPs would agree. Both parties agreed to meet in a month's time to re-evaluate the existing standards and the current process.

Follow-up

A follow-up meeting 1 month later included the primary care and hydrotherapy physiotherapists, the hospital physiotherapy manager and the general practice manager. After discussion, it was agreed that the standards would stay the same, partly as re-negotiation would need to involve all fund-holding GPs, and partly because the administration system in the hydrotherapy department had been streamlined to address the inefficiencies. The team agreed to re-audit in 6 months.

Problems can arise when one side of the interface adheres more closely to agreed standards than the other. It is always annoying when the efficiency of your own department appears to be limited by the inefficiencies of others. Here, it is vital that good communication and respect are maintained at all times. A professional approach to this type of interface peer review audit is essential in order to maintain a good working relationship. Peer review should always seek to encourage and facilitate. Apportioning blame is very easy but is unhelpful. All departments have their weaknesses and strong points. You may feel annoyed if another department appears to let you down, but you may unwittingly appear to do the same, in their view, on a different occasion – so it pays to work constructively together.

Inter-agency audit

Inter-agency audit is the evaluation of services across agency boundaries. It can occur when different agencies work together to provide services for patients and clients. For example, the NHS and Social Services work closely together to provide elderly care services, and the NHS and the Department of Education liaise to provide for children with special needs.

In some areas, purchasers buy aspects of community healthcare from voluntary or charitable agencies (e.g. in mental health). It should be remembered that the concept of clinical audit has had a number of years to become embedded within the NHS, and that this process of self-evaluation of service may be foreign to other agencies. This is not to say that other agencies do not evaluate their impact; rather, that their traditional methods of evaluation may differ by varying degrees. For example, Social Services are evaluated by quality units and the Social Services Inspectorate, and education is familiar with OFSTED and league tables. Thus, where inter-agency audit occurs, inevitably it is led by the health sector.

The National Health Service Executive, in an executive letter (NHSE, 1994), advised that the framework for clinical audit should 'promote collaborative audit between hospital, community, general practice and other agencies for example social services'. Interestingly this letter was only addressed to members of the health service, apparently encouraging an NHS lead by default.

A study of inter-agency audit involvement in the South and West Region in 1995 identified the following factors that promote the process (Barnard, 1995):

- Shared understanding of the philosophy and purpose of audit
- Commitment to collaborative audit at and between all levels of the organizations
- Absolute clarity regarding the audit topic, its aims and objectives
- Flexibility as to audit design
- A mutually acceptable and identifiable audit team, including the project manager
- An audit assistant/data gatherer who has an understanding of the culture and workings of the agencies involved in the audit and who is accepted and respected by all parties
- Ease of access to the necessary data, formally agreed if possible
- Formalized communications networks and regular joint meetings
- Training in audit for participants unfamiliar with the processes
- An allocated, agreed budget to fund the audit with clear agreement on budget-holding responsibilities.

Various problems can arise in inter-agency audit in addition to those already identified in uniprofessional, multiprofessional, and interface audits. These include:

- Imposition of audit on a reluctant team
- Lack of designated audit support
- Confusion as to the purpose and process of the audit
- Different agendas held by different agencies underlying the purpose of the audit
- Inability to agree if perceived goals and standards differ due to differing philosophies
- Lack of agreement over interpretation of the results of audit

- Problems accessing different agency records
- Steep learning curves for non-NHS staff who may be unfamiliar with audit.

However, all is not doom and gloom. Many people have found inter-agency audit to be a useful tool to improve the efficiency and effectiveness of service delivery and intervention across and between different agencies. It can lead to a smoother transition for patients or clients, less duplication of services and the plugging of gaps in service delivery that each agency thought the other was addressing. It can also have positive knock-on effects for the agencies concerned. These were identified in the South and West Region study as:

- A good opportunity to set joint goals for individual clients and service delivery
- An aid to communication between and within agencies
- A natural progression towards separate and joint service evaluation
- Better understanding of the service culture and 'language' of the other agencies.

References

Barnard S. (1995). *Whose Audit? Consumer Involvement and Inter-Agency Collaboration In Audit.* Report No. 29, ssriu, University of Portsmouth.
NHSE. (1994). *Clinical Audit: 1994/95 and Beyond.* EL(94)20: 28 February. NHSE, Leeds.

15

Involving patients, carers and their representatives in clinical audit

Patients, relatives and carers are all consumers of healthcare services. Healthy members of the population are also potential, if not existing, consumers of healthcare. Healthcare comes in many guises. Medical or other therapeutic intervention during illness or following trauma is an obvious service, but so are preventative services such as vaccination programmes, health promotion campaigns and 'Well Woman' and 'Well Man' screening clinics. Other health services providing for well populations include maternity care and family planning, school medical and dental services and child development checks. All these consumers have a vested interest in maintaining the quality, efficiency and effectiveness of health services being past, present or potentially future users.

Not all consumers of healthcare services are well enough or able to comment on the quality of service provision. This does not mean that they have no views nor that any views they have are of little value. It does mean that it may be more difficult to ascertain those views. Many consumer groups act as representatives for these people. These may be public organizations such as the community health councils run in each health authority, or action groups run by charities or voluntary organizations such as Age Concern or MIND.

Role of consumers in healthcare

The role of consumers in healthcare and other public services has received much consideration (Beresford and Croft, 1993; Croft and Beresford, 1990; Potter, 1988; Winkler, 1987). The definition of 'the consumer', the development of consumerism in healthcare, consumer representation, type of consumer involvement, and ability and access to participation are all current issues in health service management when discussing the best provision of care.

The NHS reforms over the past 10 years, based in part on the document *Working for Patients* (Department of Health, 1989) and the NHS and Community Care Act 1989, have transformed the patient from passive recipient of prescribed healthcare services to active participant in consultation with both purchasers and providers. Community health councils have represented the views of public and patient to national and local health services since 1974, but it has been the development of the internal NHS market, since the early 1990s, that has given a louder voice to the health service consumer. *The Patient's Charter* (HMSO, 1991) has spawned a myriad of local charters and practice guidelines identifying the rights of patients, but also raising consumer expectation. Before people can express an opinion about a service, they need to have experience of that service or some knowledge of it. Harrison and Wistow (1992) found that in the early days of the reforms, health service users did not always feel sufficiently educated to make choices about healthcare provision. Even in 1995 when Taylor looked at how service users' views were sought by purchasers, she found differing levels of involvement depending on the organizational development of the purchasing authority (Taylor, 1995). However, Taylor also found that some purchasers valued consumer involvement as a means to a better mutual understanding of need and resources. Dunning and Needham (1993) reported that reluctance on the part of some clinicians continues to inhibit full consumer participation in discussions on healthcare.

Types of involvement

Rigge (1995) divides consumer involvement into two categories:

1. Consultative, i.e. patients, carers and their representatives being involved in the actual consultative process, and actively involved in both discussions and policy making.
2. Participatory, i.e. patients, carers and their representatives being asked for their views (usually in a 'one-off' situation), being participants in satisfaction surveys or recipients of anonymous questionnaires.

This is true of consumer involvement in clinical audit. More often, patients are the passive participants in process or outcome audits. Consultative involvement is less common.

Consumer audit

The College of Health has a lot of experience of involving patients and their carers in consumer audit, which they define as 'a qualitative approach to obtaining feedback from patients about healthcare services; an independent, rigorous, holistic approach to obtaining consumer views' (College of Health, 1994). Consumer audit is conducted by external researchers who conduct in-depth surveys, usually in the form of focus groups or individual patient interviews. These audits provide valuable information about healthcare services but are, by their very nature, an expensive option. Consumer audits often take the form of research surveys, although it can be possible to ascertain from the analysed data whether set standards have been achieved. Kelson (1995) has produced a comprehensive report reviewing the development of consumer involvement in audit, and the literature surrounding its practice. Consumer audits published by the College of Health include Davies (1990) looking at people with a physical disability, outpatient and continence services (College of Health, 1992), services for elderly people (Bradburn, 1993) and women with breast cancer (Loughlan and Lang, 1993). The College of Health has also produced a comprehensive manual for those wishing to undertake consumer audit (College of Health, 1994) and some approaches to obtaining consumer feedback in general practice (Dennis, 1991).

Getting patients and carers involved

An executive letter in 1994, from the NHSE to NHS trusts, identified the need to 'respond to the views of local patients and patient advocacy groups' when undertaking clinical audit (NHSE, 1994).

Research by one of the authors in the South and West Region, undertaken a year after these guidelines were published, identified several factors that influence consumer involvement in audit (Barnard, 1995).

Participatory or consultative?

Many physiotherapists want to involve patients and carers in the audit process, believing that their views are vital to the full picture of service delivery evaluation. Practical involvement can be consultative or participatory (Rigge, 1995).

Consultative involvement is achieved by consideration of the following:

- Invite a patient/carer representative on to the trust audit committee
- Invite a patient/carer representative on to the audit project team in the department
- Invite a patient/carer to attend discussions about standards and patient appropriate outcomes or criteria
- Consider using a patient/carer as a data gatherer
- Consider involving a patient/carer in the data analysis process to gain a user perspective
- Enlist the help of the patient/ carer representative to feed back the results of the audit to user groups.

Participatory involvement includes some of the following:

- Use patient satisfaction questionnaires to identify topics for audit
- Use patient satisfaction surveys to audit 'patient perceived' actual

Table 15.1 Comparison of consultative and participatory involvement in clinical audit

Consultative involvement	Participatory involvement
Views of one or two representative patients/carers only	Possible to ask many people's views
Representative involved throughout audit	Patient/carer views sought in isolation
Time consuming for representative attending audit team meetings	Questionnaires quick to complete, focus groups usually a one-off
Cost implication to fund representative's expenses	Patient questionnaires relatively cheap to administer Independent focus group facilitation and feedback report expensive

practice against set standards in all types of audit (structure, process and outcome)
- Organize independently led focus groups to ascertain in-depth views about different aspects of service delivery from a group of patients/carers.

A comparison of consultative and participatory involvement in clinical audit is demonstrated in Table 15.1.

Representative user?

It is possible that the person asked to represent patients and carers will either be a willing volunteer with strong personal views or an unwilling conscript with little interest in the topic under audit. Either way, the perspective he or she brings to the team will be less than objective or representative. Issues of lay representation are well understood within the statutory health and welfare services (Taylor, 1995) which need, continually, to balance the possibility of biased consumer views against the possibility of tokenism – that is, recruiting a lay representative solely for the sake of political correctness. Recruitment of volunteers may be achieved by approaching patient panels via the trust or purchasers, by asking self-help and local charitable groups, or by displaying a notice in the departmental waiting area. The community health council may also be able to direct you towards possible volunteers. When seeking consumer representation, always consider age, sex, race, social class, and (where relevant) disability and sexual orientation.

It is not always necessary to ask patients or carers to come to you to express their views. Consider visiting a stroke group, Arthritis Care or MS Society meeting and talking with members about their experiences of your service.

Do not let the fear of tokenism or strong personal views prevent you from recruiting anyone! Remember, every clinician brings his or her personal views to the discussion table too. How representative are you of your profession or colleagues when discussing service delivery?

Confidentiality

Many clinicians express concern over the confidentiality of patient records and data used in audit, and the appropriateness of allowing lay representatives access to such material. It must be emphasized that all patient information is confidential and should not be made available to anyone not actively involved in the care of that patient. However, it is possible to include lay representatives in the organization and process of clinical audit. As long as patient data have been anonymized (according to the fundamental principles of clinical audit), or have been analysed statistically, no individual patient information is accessible. It is sensible to discuss issues of confidentiality openly with any lay representative, and to draw up a mutually agreeable code of confidentiality (including access to materials and meetings) before the audit commences.

Training lay representatives

Physiotherapists may use their own language and jargon to communicate with one another, but these might be completely incomprehensible to patients and carers. Audit terminology and its process are also new to lay representatives. Many patient/carer representatives are also new to the committee process and lack the skill or confidence to participate fully. These potential problems can be addressed by making the following arrangements:

- Give the representative full information about the audit process prior to any meetings
- Ask the purchasers and community health council whether they run training sessions for lay representatives wishing to get involved in aspects of consumer participation in local health services
- Allocate an audit team member to act as link person and befriender
- Ensure all literature is accessible, whether just jargon free or in an appropriate format to the participant's disability or culture, e.g. large print or in the participant's first language
- Avoid physiotherapy or clinical audit jargon in meetings and paperwork
- Ensure paperwork is sent out in plenty of time for the representative to ask any questions prior to meetings.

Equality of participation

In our hierarchical health service, it is easy for patients and carers to feel inferior. Lay representatives should be made welcome and assured that their views are important. It is not enough just to state this at the beginning – clinician and management commitment to this aspect of audit must be shown practically by allowing, or even prompting, the lay representatives to have their say and respecting their views. A representative may feel less confident if attending alone. Inviting two lay representatives may double the views as well as their confidence. Guidelines agreed and set down at the beginning can ensure equality of participation for all – managers, clinicians and patient/carer representatives.

Most audit meetings are held during work hours whilst clinicians are being paid their usual wage. Patients and carers, however, will doubtless be attending in their own time, possibly at their own expense and, often, at some inconvenience. Make things easier by considering the following:

- Arrange meeting times that are suitable for *all* participants
- Are child-care facilities needed?
- Are sitting services needed to allow carers to attend?
- Do you need to arrange advocacy services?
- Do you need to arrange signing or interpretation? (Client representation using Makaton sign language has been used very successfully by learning disability service providers)
- Do you need to arrange for transport for patient representatives?
- Do lay representatives need reimbursement for their expertise and time?
- Budget to plan for representative involvement.

Independent clinical auditor

There is some evidence to suggest that patients and carers are more willing to become involved in audit, either in a consultative or participatory role, if the auditors are independent of the service being audited (Kelson, 1995). This appears to reduce the anxiety that they may be discriminated against in the future as a result of their comments.

However, specialist consultants are expensive and are probably beyond departmental audit funds, although it may be worth making a case for top-up funding from the trust. It is also worth contacting your local university (School of Physiotherapy or Social Policy unit) who may be able to provide a postgraduate researcher at a reasonable cost. In-house, a non-clinical expert such as an audit facilitator may be a cheaper and more than adequate alternative.

References

Barnard S. (1995). *Whose Audit? Consumer Involvement and Inter-Agency Collaboration in Audit*. Report No. 29, Social Services Research and Information Unit, University of Portsmouth.
Beresford P. and Croft S. (1993). *Getting Involved – A Practical Manual*. Open Services Project and Joseph Rowntree Foundation, York.

Bradburn J. (1993). *South Bedfordshire Consumer Health Audit*. College of Health, London.

College of Health. (1992). *Consumer Audit: Pilot Project Report*. College of Health, London.

College of Health. (1994). *Consumer Audit Guidelines*. College of Health, London.

Croft S. and Beresford P. (1990). *From Paternalism To Participation: Involving Patients In Social Services*. Open Services Project and Joseph Rowntree Foundation, York.

Davies S. (1990). *Services for People With a Physical Disability in Parkside Health Authority*. College of Health, London.

Dennis N. (1991). *Ask The Patient: New Approaches to Consumer Feedback In General Practice*. College of Health, London.

Department of Health (1989). *Medical Audit: Working Paper 6 – Working for Patients*. HMSO, London.

Dunning M. and Needham G. (eds) (1993). *But Will it Work, Doctor?: Report of a Conference About Involving Users Of Health Services in Outcomes Research*. Kings Fund Centre, London.

Harrison S. and Wistow G. (1992). The purchaser provider split in English healthcare: towards explicit rationing. *Policy and Politics*, **20**, 123–130.

HMSO (1991). *The Patient's Charter*. HMSO, London.

Kelson M. (1995). *Consumer Involvement Initiatives in Clinical Audit and Outcomes*. College of Health, London.

Loughlan L. and Lang L. (1993). *Services For Women With Breast Cancer in West Dorset General Hospital NHS Trust*. College of Health, London.

NHSE. (1994). *Clinical Audit: 1994/5 and Beyond*. EL(94)20: 28 February. NHSE, London.

Potter J. (1988). Consumerism and the public sector: how does the coat fit? *Public Administration*, **66**, 149–164.

Rigge M. (1995). *Proceedings: South and West Regional Clinical Audit and Clinical Effectiveness Conference*. South and West Regional Health Authority, Bristol.

Taylor P. (1995). *Consumer Involvement in Health Care Commissioning*. Report No. 30, Social Services Research and Information Unit, University of Portsmouth.

Winkler F. (1987). Consumerism in healthcare: beyond the supermarket model. *Policy and Politics*, **15**, 1–8.

16
Looking towards the future

Throughout this book, we have looked at physiotherapy service evaluation through clinical audit. Already, clinical audit is becoming a well-established part of normal clinical practice throughout the National Health Service and within other healthcare providers. Clinical audit has paved the way for further service evaluation and optimization of valuable resources by encouraging critical and reflective appraisal of all aspects of clinical practice. However, there are many areas where the principles of clinical audit can be usefully employed, and this final chapter touches on some of the wider ranging issues that surround and impact on physiotherapy service provision.

Audit as a means of continuous physiotherapy service evaluation

Clinical audit is a powerful tool capable of examining all areas of a physiotherapy service from checking that all the equipment is in working order to ensuring that discharge procedures are running efficiently. Although there is some overlap between the three Donabedian categories of structure, process and outcome, it is well worth using these as a framework for setting up a rolling audit programme within the department (see Chapter 4). Senior staff should agree the topics for departmental audit on an annual basis, taking into account purchaser requirements, any new Government or trust initiatives, and any staff-generated local priorities. Plan a realistic programme by taking the following into account:

- Allow enough time to undertake the audit. It is very easy to underestimate the time required for setting up the audit and gathering all the data.
- Communicate! Ensure everyone involved knows what is going on and are, where possible, in agreement.
- Although a department may have several audits underway at once, make sure that individual units and staff are involved in only one audit at a time.

- Give staff a break between audits by running the next project within another unit.
- Ensure audits are timely: a real-life audit of physiotherapy intervention standards for patients with chronic obstructive pulmonary disease failed to gather enough data simply because it was programmed to run during the summer months when few of the patients needed hospitalization.

Continuing professional development and accreditation

Continuing professional development (CPD) is something that concerns all physiotherapists. It is the discipline of keeping up to date, of reflection on personal practice and experience, and of directing career development. It is fast becoming the linchpin of accreditation.

The principles of clinical audit may be used to evaluate personal CPD through auditing personally set standards and criteria. *The CPD Diary*, first produced by the CSP in 1992, is a useful tool for gathering evidence of personal professional development. Evidence of having achieved personal goals can be used in individual performance reviews with line managers, and as a baseline for continued professional development. Collecting evidence of CPD not only allows individuals to plan career development, but will no doubt be required in accreditation for maintenance of state registration in the future. At the time of going to press, it seems likely that evidence of CPD will be required, certainly in terms of amount (e.g. evidence of having attended a certain number of courses) and, possibly, in terms of quality (although how this will be assessed is by no means certain). It would seem sensible to keep a reflective CPD diary, with clear evidence of having achieved personally set professional goals, which can be evaluated by a quick audit in order to prepare for future accreditative procedures.

Schools of physiotherapy may offer an accreditation process to their clinical supervisors, setting standards and goals for departmental and individual accreditation. Although many of the criteria are pre-determined, there is usually scope for individual physiotherapists to provide some of their own evidence. Again, audit skills are transferable to the evaluation of these personal goals.

Benchmarking

Benchmarking is another quality tool, which can be described as the continuous process of measuring products, services and practices, or the systematic identification and spread of best practice by an organization to other parts of that organization and selected competitors.

A benchmark is an agreed criterion by which a service, product or practice can be judged. Audit standards, which reflect agreed best practice, can be employed as part of these criteria. This is especially true of organizational (structure) audit standards. As more agencies compete to provide services, commissioners of healthcare will no doubt make increasing use of benchmarking surveys to inform their contracting decisions.

Clinical guidelines

In 1996, the NHSE set out its recommendations for the 'development, application and appraisal' of clinical guidelines (NHSE, 1996), in which clinical guidelines were described as 'systematically developed statements which assist clinicians and patients in making decisions about appropriate treatment for specific conditions'. It was emphasized that the responsibility for development, publication and maintenance of guidelines remains with the appropriate professional body. Physiotherapists are taking up this challenge with national specific interest groups developing clinical guidelines for physiotherapy intervention in their field.

Guidelines are drawn up based on firm evidence from research findings and clinical experience through consensus (Eccles et al., 1996). The NHSE recommends that clinical guidelines should not only be appraised by appropriate experts, in the light of research evidence, but monitored, whilst in use, through the clinical audit process.

The last word

As we have seen, clinical audit has evolved exponentially since its tenuous introduction into healthcare in 1989. Its role may continue to change and evolve both with future Government initiatives and as clinicians find new areas where this valuable tool can be employed, but the principles of clinical audit are now firmly embedded within National Health Service culture and need to be learned and understood by all professional groups. We hope that this book will assist physiotherapists as they embark upon clinical audit, perhaps for the first time, and that it will be used as a resource to expand the collective physiotherapy experience of clinical audit.

References

Eccles M., Clapp Z., Grimshaw J., Adam P.C., Higgins B., Purves I., Russell I. (1996). Developing valid guidelines: methodological and procedural issues from the North of England Evidence Based Guideline Development Project. *Quality in Health Care*, 5, 44–50.
NHSE (1996). *Clinical Guidelines – Using Clinical Guidelines to Improve Patient Care Within the NHS*. Crown Copyright. NHSE, Leeds.

Useful addresses

Senior Professional Advisor (Clinical Audit)
Chartered Society of Physiotherapy
14 Bedford Row
London WC1R 4ED
Tel: 0171 306 6633

Cochrane Library is available from:

BMJ Publishing Group
PO Box 295
London WC1H 9TE
Tel: 0171 383 6185/6245

College of Health
St. Margaret's House
21 Old Ford Road
London E2 9PL
Tel: 0181 983 1553

National Centre for Clinical Audit (NCCA)
BMA House
Tavistock Square
London WC1H 9JP
Tel: 0171 383 6451

NHS Centre for Reviews and Dissemination
Information Service
Heslington
York YO1 5DD
Tel: 01904 433707

TELER®
PO Box 699
Sheffield S17 3YG
Tel: 0114 236 9544

UK Clearing House for the Information on the Assessment of Health Outcomes
Nuffield Institute for Health
71–75 Clarendon Road
Leeds LS2 9PL
Tel: 0113 233 3940

Index